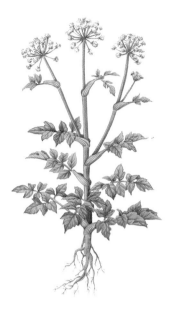

HEALTH AND HEALING
THE NATURAL WAY

NATURE'S
MEDICINE CHEST

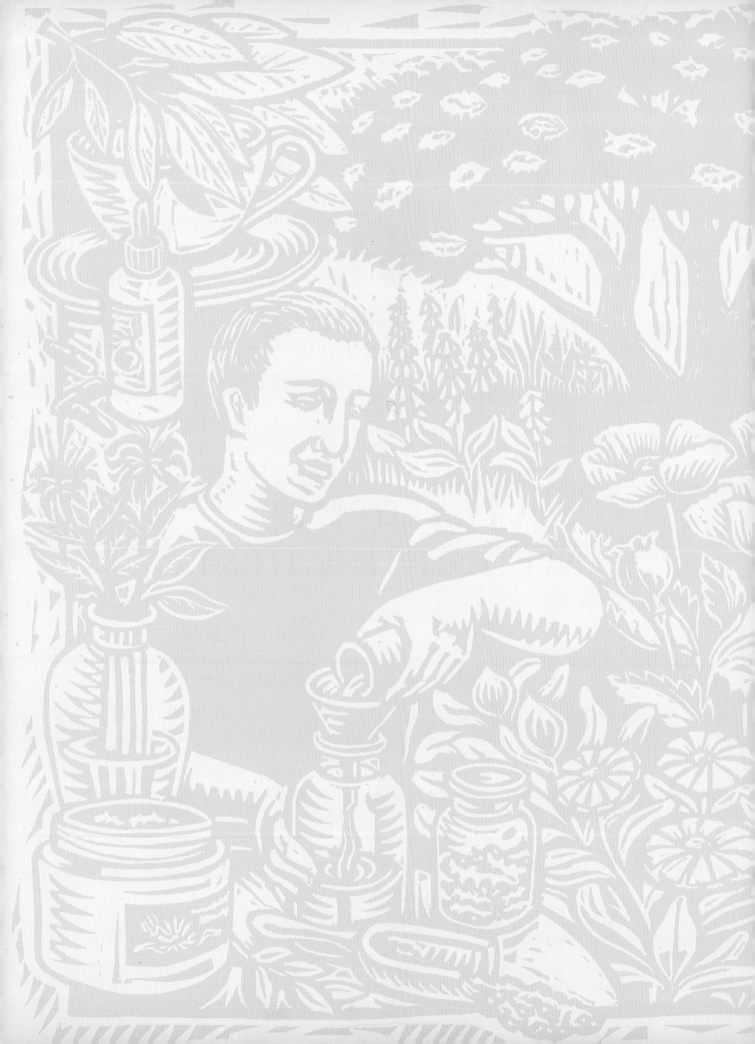

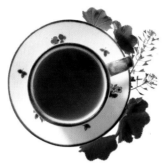

Health And Healing
The Natural Way

Nature's Medicine Chest

PUBLISHED BY
THE READER'S DIGEST ASSOCIATION, INC.
PLEASANTVILLE, NEW YORK / MONTREAL

A READER'S DIGEST BOOK
Produced by
Carroll & Brown Limited, London

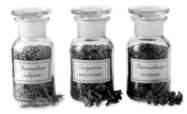

CARROLL & BROWN

Publishing Director Denis Kennedy
Art Director Chrissie Lloyd

Managing Editor Sandra Rigby
Managing Art Editor Tracy Timson

Editor Laura Price

Art Editor Gilda Pacitti
Designers Rachel Goldsmith, Jonathan Wainwright

Photographers David Murray, Jules Selmes

Production Wendy Rogers, Clair Reynolds

Computer Management John Clifford, Karen Kloot

First English Edition Copyright © 1997
The Reader's Digest Association Limited,
11 Westferry Circus, Canary Wharf,
London E14 4HE

Printed in the United States of America

ISBN 0-7621-0261-6

Library of Congress cataloging in publication data
has been applied for.

CONSULTANT

Christopher Hedley MNIMH
Medical Herbalist

CONTRIBUTORS

Julian Barker Dip. Phyt., MNIMH
Medical Herbalist

Mark Evans MNIMH
Medical Herbalist

Adrian McDermott BSc., MNIMH
Medical Herbalist

Sabine Rickert MNIMH
Medical Herbalist

FOR READER'S DIGEST

Project Editor Gayla Visalli

READER'S DIGEST GENERAL BOOKS

Editor in Chief, U.S. General Books Christopher Cavanaugh
Editorial Director, health & medicine Wayne Kalyn
Design Director, health & medicine Barbara Rietschel

READER'S DIGEST BOOKS & HOME ENTERTAINMENT, CANADA

Vice President and Editorial Director Deirdre Gilbert
Managing Editor Philomena Rutherford
Art Director John McGuffie

The information in this book is for reference only;
it is not intended as a substitute for a doctor's diagnosis and care.
The editors urge anyone with continuing medical problems
or symptoms to consult a doctor.

NATURE'S MEDICINE CHEST

More and more people today are choosing to take greater responsibility for their own health rather than relying on the doctor to step in with a cure when something goes wrong. We now recognize that we can influence our health by making certain improvements in lifestyle—eating better, doing more exercise, and taking measures to reduce stress. People are also becoming increasingly aware that there are other healing methods—some new, others ancient—that can help prevent illness or be used as complements to orthodox medicine.

The series *Health and Healing the Natural Way* can help you make your own health choices by giving you clear, comprehensive, straightforward, and encouraging information and advice about methods of improving your health. The series explains the many different natural therapies now available, including aromatherapy, herbalism, acupressure, and a number of others, as well as the circumstances in which they benefit you when used in conjunction with conventional medicine.

NATURE'S MEDICINE CHEST introduces you to the diverse and fascinating realm of herbalism. It provides a clear and concise guide to the ways in which herbal preparations can help to relieve and heal common health problems. The book is filled with information on how to prepare and apply herbal remedies and tells you which particular ones are recommended for specific complaints—from arthritis to the common cold. You will also find a fascinating overview of ancient herbal wisdom and learn how herbalism is being practiced today, as well as which herbal remedies have been scientifically verified through numerous studies. At the heart of the book is a fully illustrated A-to-Z guide to many widely used healing herbs, with notes on dosage and preparations and any special cautions. *NATURE'S MEDICINE CHEST* shows you how easy it is to bring the benefits of herbal remedies into your life.

CONTENTS

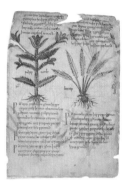

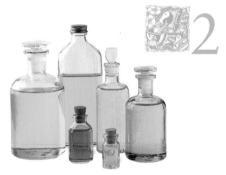
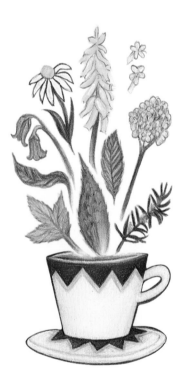

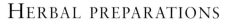

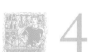

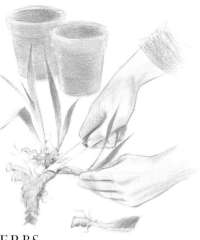
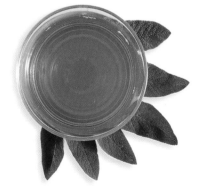

HERBAL HEALING

Insight into the age-old traditions of herbal remedies can help you to enjoy the powerful medicinal value of plants.

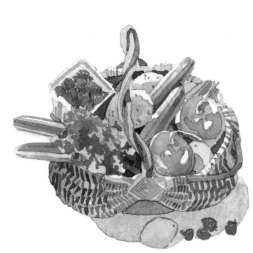

CULINARY MEDICINES
Many staple foods have medicinal benefits as well, though these are not obtained necessarily through ingestion. Cabbage leaves and potato juice can both be used as poultices to relieve swelling and tenderness. Other plants that bring relief include strawberries for sunburn, cucumber for itchy skin, and onion for bee stings.

EGYPTIAN HEALING
References to herbal remedies, some still used today, have been found in ancient Egyptian texts.

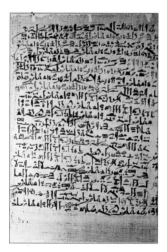

Herbs were recorded in the earliest writings, and they have played a part in the evolution of human societies all over the world. The ancient Egyptians used herbs for many purposes, and the Bible refers to herbs such as frankincense and myrrh being used cosmetically and medicinally. North American shamans have used herbs in their healing, as have the Chinese, Persians, Aborigines of Australia, and other peoples. However, orthodox medical practitioners in the Western world are only just beginning to recognize the real medicinal value of many common herbs.

Despite the growing importance of herbalism today, there appears to be no single definition of an herb. Some definitions focus on the medicinal properties of the plant, and others on culinary uses. Nevertheless, it seems that most people agree that an herb is a plant, all or parts of which are used as a medicine, a flavoring for food, and/or an aromatic or chemical addition to cosmetics. Such a definition, however, opens the term *herbalism* to a great many geographical and social interpretations.

HERBALISM THROUGHOUT HISTORY

For most of history and for the majority of the world's cultures, there has been no strict delineation between plants that were used for healing and those that were used for food. All societies lived off the land, and a variety of local plants made up part of their diet. It is hardly surprising, therefore, that people everywhere discovered medical uses for their local flora.

Around the world healers have worked with a whole range of herbal preparations, endeavoring to treat any illness that presented itself. Inevitably, some of these early treatments proved to be ineffective and even dangerous, yet many survived to the present day and are still recommended because they are beneficial.

One of the earliest extant records of herbal medicine, the Ebers Papyrus (named for the German Egyptologist Georg Ebers), is believed to have been written in the 16th century B.C. It contains more than 700 references to herbs, many of which are still used today. Other peoples, most notably the Aztecs, North American Indians, and Persians, understood the medicinal value of herbs as long ago as 1000 B.C.

In Europe the Greeks and Romans furthered the ancient knowledge of herbal remedies, and much of their learning survived unaltered into the Middle Ages. The advent of the printing press brought with it the first medical and herbal books, which were among the earliest books to be printed, and until the 16th century, herbalism was by far the most widely practiced form of healing and medicine in Europe.

WITCHCRAFT AND THE DECLINE OF HERBALISM

Healers have always held a position of power in society, whether those societies were primitive or sophisticated. Many healers practiced herbalism to a greater or lesser degree and were renowned and respected for their herbal knowledge.

Despite this fact, many 16th- and 17th-century female healers and midwives were singled out for persecution during the famous witch hunts of those eras. This could possibly be attributed to their use of herbal preparations. Many herbs that were widely used for medicinal purposes were also thought to be part of occult rituals. If the healer's potions and concoctions did not succeed as cures, they might have been viewed as poisons or deliberate acts of ill will.

Even the harvesting of herbs was believed to change the plants' powers for good or evil. Some herbs used for their medicinal properties were picked during a full moon to improve their healing powers. Those used in witchcraft were supposedly more powerful for malignant purposes when harvested as the moon waned. Some of the most poisonous herbs known were believed to have been used in the witches' potions for flying and were therefore seen as strongly related to mysticism and the forces of evil.

Herbs also played a protective role in superstitious beliefs, however, and not every herbalist and healer suffered at the hands of the witch hunters. Rue (*Ruta graveolens*) was believed to hinder acts of witchcraft and diminish the potency of spells and hexes, while garlic (*Allium sativum*) is a well-documented protection

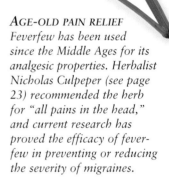

AGE-OLD PAIN RELIEF
Feverfew has been used since the Middle Ages for its analgesic properties. Herbalist Nicholas Culpeper (see page 23) recommended the herb for "all pains in the head," and current research has proved the efficacy of feverfew in preventing or reducing the severity of migraines.

WITCHES' BREW
Witchcraft, magic, and healing have long been associated. For centuries potions and preparations have been equated with the summoning of spirits, the capturing of souls, and the power of flight.

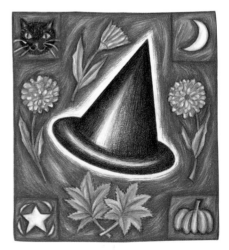

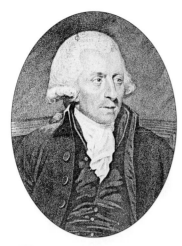

ACTIVE PLANT MATERIALS
Research into the effects of plants on the body has led to the use of many plant remedies, such as nasturtium leaves, a natural antibiotic.

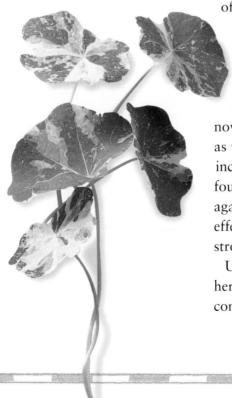

against vampires. When the terror of the witch hunts waned, there developed a more scientific and less superstitious approach to the art of healing and the power of herbs.

MODERN HERBALISM

The move from traditional folklore toward a more scientific approach to herbs was aided by a growth in chemical and botanical understanding and advances in the tools used for analysis. This change began early in the 19th century, and many herbalists consider that it started in earnest with the discovery of how to extract essential elements from plants, for instance, quinine from the cinchona tree. With these advances, scientists began to explore the effects that plant-based chemicals had on the human body while at the same time trying to identify the microorganisms that invade the body and cause diseases such as malaria. These two areas of research came together as herbal properties were employed in the battle against disease, and knowledge of the medicinal value of plants finally began to find its place in the medicine of the day.

In 1785 the English physician William Withering discovered the positive effects that foxglove (*Digitalis purpurea*) had on heart failure. He examined local herbalists' claims that foxglove leaves would cure dropsy—water retention—and recognized dropsy as a symptom of heart disease. His experiments showed that the foxglove did indeed relieve the effects of heart failure. Today one of the most potent and widely used heart stimulants, digoxin, is derived from the foxglove.

HERBS UNDER THE MICROSCOPE

The chemical analysis of plant matter throughout the 20th century has revealed a number of active constituents that we now know are responsible for the physiological effects of herbal, as well as many conventional, remedies. These active ingredients, including vitamins, minerals, saponins, and tannins, have all been found to affect various parts of the body, thus helping to protect against or bring relief from many disorders. Tannins, for example, effectively draw the cells of the skin together and thus create a stronger barrier against infection.

Using this knowledge of the effects of herbal ingredients allows herbalists to apply specific herbal remedies to disorders in relative confidence of the outcome.

As a form of healing, herbalism has gained growing respect among practitioners of conventional medicine and among those who have benefited from herbal treatment, and its popularity is now established throughout the world.

PROFESSIONAL HERBALISM

In the past 60 years the role of the professional herbalist has grown in the Western world. Although some 25 percent of prescription drugs and more than 50 percent of over-the-counter medicines have active constituents derived from plants, their formulations are often harsher and have more potential side effects than natural plant products. With improvements in the chemical industry that make it possible for herbal extracts to be purer and more accessible than before, the popularity of over-the-counter herbal remedies in the West continues to grow.

An herbalist believes in a holistic approach to healing—treating the cause of an illness and the person as a whole rather than just the symptoms of the disease—and therefore needs to study a patient in some detail to prescribe precisely those herbs that will give the most benefit. Professional herbalists also give detailed advice to the individual with regard to curing and relieving general health problems, as well as information on herbs and their actions.

Although a professional herbalist has access to more herbs and more detailed information than a person attempting self-treatment, the growing respect for herbalism has increased the interest in and availability of self-help remedies. (Chapters 2 through 6 of this book can help you identify many common medicinal plants and prepare your own remedies with them.)

HERBS AND HEALTH

Most herbal remedies are simple to make and to apply. Both internal remedies, such as teas, tinctures, and syrups, and external applications, like compresses, poultices, creams, and ointments, can usually be prepared at home with basic kitchen equipment. Depending on which parts of a plant are used, the active ingredients, and how it is prepared, a remedy can have different effects on the body and on particular ailments. It does not necessarily follow that different preparations of an herb will be equally useful, so when treating yourself, always monitor both your symptoms and your remedies.

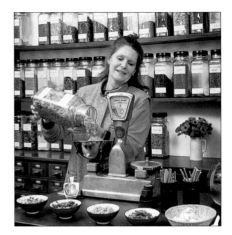

HERBALISM TODAY
Modern herbalists have gained recognition in the West, and medicinal herbs are now sold freely in the United Kingdom, Europe, and North America.

HOME HEALING
The increased interest in herbalism and the greater amount of information available have led to many people making and applying herbal remedies at home.

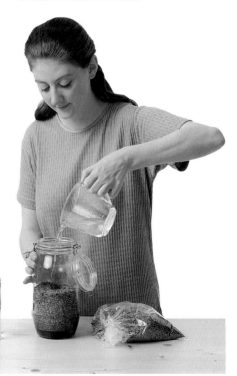

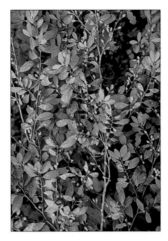

COCA PLANT
Many plants have specific chemical derivatives that alter bodily functions. One of the most widely known is the illegal stimulant cocaine, derived from the coca plant.

KITCHEN CURES
Most herbal preparations are easy to prepare and to use. Honeysuckle syrup is a home remedy that offers fast and effective relief from sore throats.

HOW TO USE THIS BOOK

The purpose of NATURE'S MEDICINE CHEST is to unravel and expose both the facts and the fiction of herbal healing. Chapter 1 offers a working definition of medicinal plants throughout history and looks at herbs as drugs, as well as foods. It surveys age-old remedies from around the world and reveals how the pharmaceutical industry evolved from the study of plants. The chapter then explores some of the pharmaceutical preparations made from herbs today and highlights the differences between herbal remedies and other drugs in preparation, action, and use.

In Chapter 2 the current use of herbs in various therapies, from herbalism to homeopathy, and in the make-up of household products is discussed. The growth of herbalism underscores the importance of the rain forests of South America and their vast wealth of untapped healing. A brief look at genetic engineering and the role it plays in finding new natural medicines and "designing" plants with higher quantities of healing properties concludes the chapter, along with a glance at the future of herbal remedies.

Using herbs safely is an important part of home herbalism. In Chapter 3 you will learn how to find and prepare herbs, where to buy or pick them, and how to assess their quality. You will also learn how to store herbs to keep them fresh and how to prepare remedies without destroying the herbs' therapeutic properties. Here, too, you will find out about the properties of different parts of a plant, discover which ones are best for home use and which are unsafe, and learn about the dangers of self-diagnosis and overdosing.

If you'd rather grow, harvest, dry, and prepare your own herbs, Chapter 4 gives all the advice you need—from planning a garden to applying your homemade cream. In Chapter 5 you will find more than 85 common medicinal herbs listed in alphabetical order under their Latin names. Each entry includes a botanical description of the herb with its history, active ingredients, recommendations for use, and, when necessary, cautions and contraindications. Illnesses that respond well to herbal self-treatment are discussed in Chapter 6, where you will find all the information you need for relieving many common ailments. If you have a disorder and wish to use herbs to treat it, you can turn straight to Chapter 6 for proven remedies.

WHAT ARE HERBAL REMEDIES?

Many plants contain substances that affect the body's systems. When these plant extracts are used to treat illness or disease, the treatment is deemed an herbal remedy. To use herbal remedies to their best effect, it is important to understand the nature of the remedies and to make and apply them safely.

Q **WHERE DID HERBAL MEDICINE COME FROM?**
No one can truly answer this question because one of the oldest uses of herbs yet discovered dates back to prehistoric times. It is possible to state, however, that herbalism is thousands of years old and has been used by the most advanced and creative civilizations ever known. For many people the term *herbalism* may conjure up images of Druids or witches concocting magic potions, undermining any belief in the medicinal efficacy of the remedies themselves. In the past century the claims made for herbs in healing have come under increased scientific scrutiny, and an amazing number of remedies have been proved effective.

In Chapter 1 you will find a wide-ranging history of the medicinal use of herbs, details on their current uses, scientific progress that is being made in the advancement of herbalism, and a glance at the future of healing with herbs. Chapter 2 focuses on the use of herbal preparations in various healing therapies, such as aromatherapy and massage, and the many common products that contain herbal extracts.

Q **HOW DO HERBAL REMEDIES WORK?**
The plants that are most widely used in herbal remedies contain many active therapeutic constituents that act upon the body. Such actions, whether gently toning skin or causing sudden vomiting, can be harnessed and applied to relieve acute illness and chronic disease. Some herbs have been used medicinally for thousands of years, but the extent of their therapeutic use may only recently have come to light. Echinacea, for example, has long been used to fight infections such as colds and flu, but current research into its immune-system-boosting effects has raised hopes that it may prove useful in the treatment of HIV and AIDS. For information on the active constituents of herbs and the physiological effects these have in fighting disease, see Chapters 4 and 5.

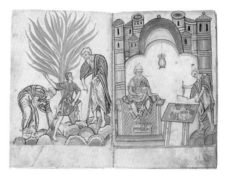

HERBAL HISTORY
Early herbals, such as Dioscorides' famous book, De Materia Medica, *help us to understand the widespread history of herbalism.*

FUTURE HERBAL REMEDIES
The flowers of hawthorn are currently being researched for their therapeutic effects in relieving heart problems.

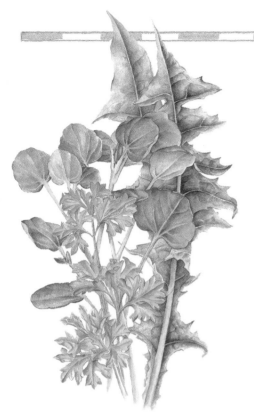

SUPER SALADS
It is recommended that some herbs be taken regularly even when you are not ill, such as those that are rich in iron and vitamins. These include salad herbs, such as watercress, parsley, and dandelion.

TEA TONIC
Drinking a cup of warm skullcap tea three times a day can help to relieve and reduce the severity of headaches.

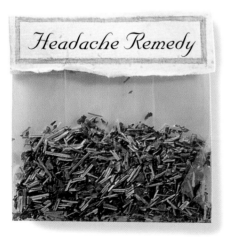

Q **WHY WOULD YOU SEE AN HERBALIST RATHER THAN A DOCTOR?**

The simple answer is that you would not. Few therapists would ever suggest that you discard the help and advice of your doctor and turn solely to herbalism to cure ills. This is not because they doubt the efficacy of the treatments, but the more complete treatment a person receives, the better. Most herbalists recommend that a general practitioner be kept informed of herbal treatments, and some will even work with your doctor to provide the most effective treatment. There are, of course, certain disorders and situations for which professional medical treatment should always be sought. For details on such disorders, see Chapter 3.

Q **IS HERBAL MEDICINE SAFE?**

Natural herbal remedies are widely considered to be less harmful to the body than chemical drugs and tend to have a gentler yet equally effective action. With any treatment, however, it is vital that you understand the limits of the actions. There are several highly toxic herbs, and even those not considered poisonous should still be taken with caution. Overdosing on herbal remedies is quite possible, and certain treatments are deemed unsafe for some people. The diversity of actions a single herb can have means that while some people may take the remedy quite safely for indigestion, others, such as a pregnant woman or someone with hypertension, may experience dangerous side effects. It is important, therefore, to be aware of the cautions and contraindications and to follow any guidelines carefully. Details for the safe application of herbal remedies can be found in Chapter 3 and in the individual entries in Chapter 5.

Q **WHAT DISORDERS CAN HERBAL REMEDIES TREAT?**

The majority of disorders an herbalist is asked to treat tend to be chronic rather than acute. This may be because many people feel more confident treating acute infections like tonsillitis with antibiotics. In fact, herbal remedies are just as effective as many synthetic drugs, and many help the body to heal itself rather than just counteracting the symptoms of an illness or disorder. Apart from the occasions, listed in Chapter 3, when herbal remedies are not advised, there are numerous disorders that an herbalist can treat effectively. In Chapter 6 you will find a number of ailments, afflicting all parts of the body, that respond well to herbal remedies and that you can make and apply at home.

CHAPTER 1

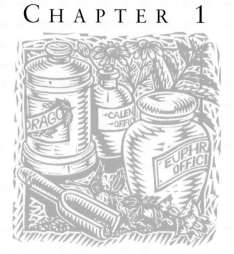

THE CURATIVE POWER OF HERBS

*Herbs and other plants have been used to
alleviate and cure illnesses since prehistoric times.
Advances in medical and scientific knowledge have
proved the efficacy of many traditional plant
remedies, some of which are at the forefront
of conventional medicine today.*

DEFINING MEDICINAL PLANTS

Strictly speaking, an herb is a plant that has no woody parts, but what we call an herbal remedy may be derived from any part of either an herbaceous or a woody plant.

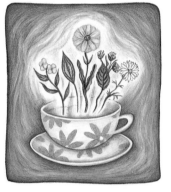

TEA THERAPY
Steeping herbs to make a tea is one of the most popular ways of using them medicinally.

Botanists use the term *herb* to describe a seed-bearing plant that has little or no woody tissue and dies down at the end of a growing season. This description differentiates it from a woody plant, that is, a tree or a shrub. But in herbal medicine the word *herb* refers to any type of vegetation and any part of it—roots, flowers, leaves, stems, fruit, bark—that is used medicinally. Other natural substances like honey are often included in the category of herbal medicine as well.

HERBS AS DRUGS AND HERBS AS FOODS

It is difficult to draw an absolute line between medicinal plants and those used for food and other purposes. If you pour boiling water on the fermented leaves of *Camellia sinensis*, you usually do so because you enjoy the taste of the resulting drink and feel better for sipping it. You are, in fact, making a cup of tea—a domestic and often social event that most people would say has nothing to do with medicine. We may not call the cup of tea medicine, but the boiling water extracts chemicals from the plant material that produce the welcome effect on the body. And this method, pouring boiling water over fresh or dried parts of a plant and steeping it to extract the beneficial constituents, is one of the most common ways of using herbs medicinally.

Many people enjoy chamomile tea, made from the plant's flowers (or a chamomile tea bag), for its taste. Few people consider its medicinal properties. If you have eaten too well or too late in the evening, a chamomile infusion can soon ease your discomfort and may also promote a restful night's sleep.

Fennel can be used to relieve indigestion, gas, and nausea.

Marjoram acts as a circulatory stimulant and helps to relieve circulation problems.

Parsley can be chewed to help combat bad breath.

CULINARY CURES
Few people are aware of the therapeutic effects of many common kitchen herbs. With proper caution, the same herb you use to flavor dishes when cooking can be used in a more concentrated form to relieve pain or lift your mood.

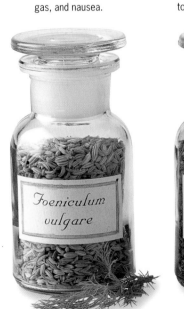
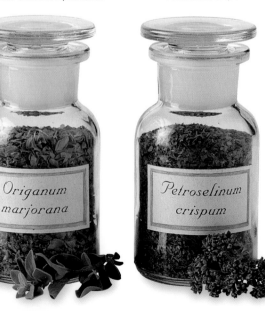

Foeniculum vulgare

Origanum marjorana

Petroselinum crispum

There are many other herbs commonly used to flavor food that also have medicinal properties. Examples are parsley, basil, mint, marjoram, oregano, rosemary, and thyme. They happen to aid digestion and may also contribute in a small way to the nutritional quality of the meal. But there is no nutritional advantage in taking large quantities. In fact, if you ate the same amount of these herbs as of potatoes, for example, you would be at risk of being poisoned. In between the culinary amount and the toxic dose lies a useful medicinal dose.

Numerous foods, besides being nutritious, are efficacious for various disorders as well. Dandelion leaves, for instance, are a vegetable that is loaded with vitamins A and C, while the root of the plant is a diuretic that can help reduce hypertension and relieve urinary infections, among other effects.

Many foods can also act medicinally when applied topically. Raw cabbage leaves, for example, help to relieve swollen arthritic joints, and cabbage juice has been found to stimulate the digestive enzymes of the stomach. Raw potatoes, likewise, make a useful poultice, and provided they have no green discoloration, the consumption of their juice can ease stomach pain.

It is interesting to note that parts of the potato plant other than the tuber are poisonous and have no therapeutic value. And a few of the potato's close relatives—deadly nightshade, henbane, and thorn apple—are all poisonous plants.

PHYTOMEDICINALS

While the medicinal value of some herbs can be experienced by eating them, others need their properties extracted with solvents. The resulting pharmaceutical preparations are called phytomedicinals—from the Greek for plant, or botanical, medicines.

Although some medicinal herbs, like feverfew, are effective in their fresh state, the majority are used dried. The process of drying herbs concentrates them and strengthens their effect. It also preserves them and makes them easier to store.

Solvents

Once an herb has been dried, a solvent must be used to extract the active ingredients. One of the most commons solvents is water. A great many botanical constituents dissolve only in water, which is the reason that so many herbs are used in the form of infusions, decoctions, or inhalants.

Another common solvent is alcohol. Many plant constituents will not dissolve in anything under 25 percent alcohol, and much higher percentages of alcohol are needed to dissolve resins (found, for example, in marigolds). The use of alcohol will vary depending on the intended application. If marigold is being used for its wound-healing properties, an extract from the plant will be made using 90 percent alcohol. To treat influenza, however, an herbalist would not use alcohol at all because the antiviral constituents are water soluble.

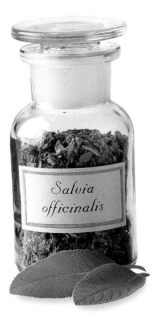
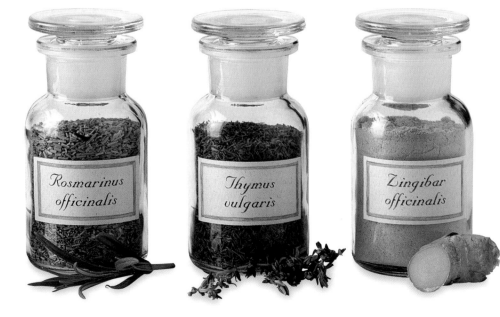

Sage has antiseptic properties and makes an effective gargle for a sore throat.

Rosemary is a warming circulatory stimulant that can lift mood and relieve fatigue.

Thyme has an expectorant action and can be used to relieve chesty coughs.

Ginger is a strong circulatory stimulant with anti-inflammatory and anticoagulant actions.

Salvia officinalis

Rosmarinus officinalis

Thymus vulgaris

Zingibar officinalis

SOME TRUTHS ABOUT HEALING HERBS

It is a fallacy that herbs cannot harm, only heal. Strychnine—one of the most highly poisonous plants and long used as an arrow poison—was once considered an effective painkiller. However, because a tiny dose can be fatal and there is no known antidote for it, strychnine is considered too deadly for general medicinal use.

It is also not necessarily true that all natural herbs are superior to synthetic drugs. Although herbs tend to have a gentler action, they may also contain impurities. Treatment of stomach ulcers using licorice may produce side effects such as hypertension because it contains glycyrrhizin. However, a useful licorice-based ulcer drug causes no side effects because the glycyrrhizin has been removed.

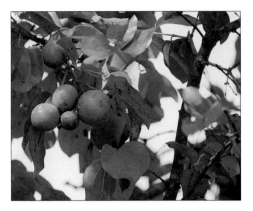

STRYCHNINE
Strychnine (Strychnos toxifera) *is one of the most poisonous plants in the world. It contains alkaloids that cause paralysis of the central nervous system, and the lethal dose is extremely small. All parts of the plant are extremely poisonous.*

Glycerol and propylene glycol are sometimes used for medicines in cases where the presence of even a small quantity of alcohol is deemed undesirable. They have their limitations as to solubility, however, and may also hinder absorption of the herbal constituents within the body.

Other solvents used in the industrial production of medicines include acetone, ether, and chloroform, which must be removed before the herbal extract can be sold.

DIFFERENCES BETWEEN HERBS AND OTHER DRUGS

Although herbs are the basis of many drugs, there is a clear difference between the way an herbalist views an herb and a pharmacist looks at a drug. An herb, in the sense that herbalists use the word, is whole-plant material—fresh, dried, or extracted. The material may be from leaves, flowers, fruits, seeds, stems, or underground organs such as roots, rhizomes, corms, or bulbs. It can also be a product like a volatile oil, obtained by distilling plant parts, or a substance exuded by the living plant, such as juice, gum, latex, or other resinous material, usually from the bark of a tree. Just one herb alone consists of many active ingredients, and herbalists often prescribe complex mixtures of herbs.

A drug, in the sense that pharmacists—and, for that matter, the general public—use

the word, often is a single compound with well-defined therapeutic goals, though some drug preparations, in fact, contain a combination of two or three drugs. Besides the active chemical itself, a preparation often contains such fillers (usually listed as inactive ingredients) as chalk or lactose, which have no therapeutic action but may aid in absorption or mask unpleasant tastes.

Many drugs are presented in a form to be swallowed (tablet, capsule, syrup), applied to the skin (cream, lotion, ointment), or introduced into a cavity of the body (eardrops, suppositories). Herbal preparations also take most of these forms, but in addition they are often administered as teas, decoctions, poultices, and inhalants (see pages 75 to 80).

HERBAL PAINKILLER
The opium poppy has been used for centuries as a painkiller and is still one of the most effective analgesics known.

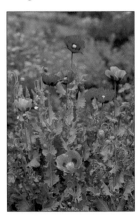

DID YOU KNOW?
Some people believe that whole herbs are generally more effective than the constituents isolated from them and used in medications. However, two of the most widely used and reliable heart-stimulant drugs, digoxin and digitoxin, are more potent than the foxglove leaf from which they are extracted, a fact that is true of many herb-based pharmaceutical drugs.

MEDICINAL PLANTS THROUGHOUT HISTORY

In all places where humans have lived, there have been healing plants too. We know of no human society in which plants have not been used to promote health and treat illness.

One of the earliest known uses of plants other than as food was discovered at a Neanderthal burial site in northern Iraq, where the remains of a man interred in flowers were unearthed in 1975. Carbon dating estimates that the burial took place some 60,000 years ago, and seven of the eight plants discovered at that site are still in use today.

Clay tablets dating from about 4000 B.C. reveal that the Sumerians had apothecaries for dispensing medicinal herbs. Primitive civilizations around the world, such as those in Papua New Guinea and the Amazon jungle, have an intimate knowledge of the plants that surround them and upon which they depend for food, medicine, clothing, and shelter. Many herbal remedies they use today were possibly used by their Stone Age forefathers. These ancient uses of plants and the fact that herbal remedies are still used worldwide today give some insight into the importance of plant life to man's existence from earliest times.

THE LEGENDARY HEALERS

Most civilizations have had healers of renown, whether real or mythological, occurrences that span centuries and continents and link the power and fame of the healers with the growth of their societies. Imhotep, the first recorded Egyptian healer, was physician to the pharaoh Zoser just under 5,000 years ago. It is difficult to separate his powers of astrology and magic from his use of plants, but his ability to heal has remained in the legends of that country for millennia. The ancient Greco-Roman god of healing, Aesculapius, may actually have lived as a man before becoming a deity. The maxim "First the word, then the herb . . .

and only then the knife" is ascribed to him. His daughter, Hygeia, was the Greek goddess of health.

The ancient Greek physician Hippocrates, perhaps the most famous healer of all and still known as the Father of Medicine, paid great attention to the medicinal use of herbs, as well as to other factors such as diet, exercise, and hygiene, in promoting health and preventing disease. The Hippocratic corpus, which laid out Hippocrates' code of medicinal practice, was written between 400 and 500 B.C. After hippocrates came Aristotle, whose far-ranging scientific work included an effort to catalog the properties of the various medicinal herbs.

The East

The earliest existing record from Eastern herbalism is the famed Chinese classical pharmacopeia, *Tzu-I Pên Tshao Ching*, thought to have been composed in China about 500 B.C. However, it is based on the

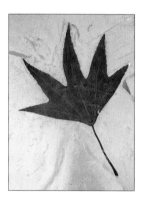

PREHISTORIC HERBS
Archeological sites all over the world have yielded fossils of plants, such as the Eocene era leaf above, found in the state of Utah. These fossils help us trace the development of plant life to the present day.

Herbal Myths

Mistletoe was once believed to grow where lightning had struck an oak tree. Druids saw mistletoe as the female essence to the oak's male principle, which may have led to its symbolism of sexuality and fertility, which lingers today in the Christmas tradition of kissing beneath it.

work of a man who lived much earlier, the legendary emperor Shen Nung, who died about 2700 B.C. The book contained nearly 300 herbs and described remedies that had been in use possibly for thousands of years.

Compilation of the *Susruta-Samhita*, the oldest medical text of India, coincided with the life of Buddha (560–480 B.C.). It names over 700 medicinal plants, arranged according to the condition to be treated. It is apparent, however, that the medicinal use of herbs was a well-established practice in India long before the creation of this text.

In the Middle East, Crateuas (120–163 B.C.) was the physician and herb collector to Mithridates, the ruler of Pontus. This herbalist-king was obsessed with the fear of being poisoned and focused much of his research on medicinal plants in the study of poisons and the search for antidotes.

The Old Testament era

Many herbs and plants mentioned in the Bible are particularly noted for medicinal use and religious observation. In Psalm 51, for example, you can find the words "Purge me with hyssop and I shall be clean." The

DID YOU KNOW?

Herbal concoctions and potions have not always been used to heal. In ancient Greece, for example, capital punishment was carried out using a draft of poisonous hemlock, which the prisoner was forced to drink. One of the most famous victims of this punishment was the Greek philosopher Socrates (469–399 B.C.).

Hebrew word *ezob* in the original text is traditionally translated as hyssop, an aromatic plant believed to have medicinal properties, and it is almost certain that purification in the religious and medical senses were not distinct. Other scholars argue that the psalmist had a marjoram in mind—one closely related to the plant used today for upper respiratory infections.

Another example can be seen in Exodus 30:34: "And the Lord said unto Moses, take unto thee sweet spices, stacte and onycha and galbanum: And thou shall make . . . a confection after the art of the apothecary, tempered together, pure and holy." Stacte is

Herbal time line

This time line illustrates the steady, worldwide interest in herbs for the past 60,000 years. Here you can trace the growth of herbal discovery from pre-historic man to the beginning of modern herbalism.

c. 60,000 B.C.
Neanderthal man buried with herbal tributes. Pollen analysis of the flowers chosen for a Neanderthal burial site in northern Iraq revealed nearly all of them to be still in use today. They included yarrow (*Alchemilla millefolium*), mallow, and grape hyacinth.

millefolium

2700 B.C.
Imhotep (above), the earliest recorded Egyptian physician, promoted carob, date, fig, olive, peach, pomegranate, garlic, lotus, and lettuce as healthy foods with medicinal uses.

2500 B.C.
The earliest Sumerian herbal written. Almonds, apricot, poppy, turmeric, sesame, and myrrh were all respected medicines. Their names were taken from the Sumerian into modern languages, indicating the great age of their use.

1500 B.C.
Advanced civilizations based upon the agriculture of corn, peppers, squash, and beans, and with an extensive use of medicinal plants, flourished in Central America and Peru.

1500 B.C.
The Egyptian Ebers Papyrus presented a written compilation of prescriptions, most of them of plant origin, arranged according to the condition to be treated.

1000 B.C.
Asklepios, or Aesculapius, the Greek mythological hero who was the god of healing, may have lived as a celebrated herbalist and healer.

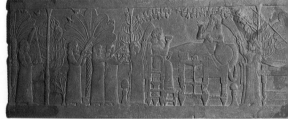

600 B.C.
Babylonian tablets (above), found in the ruins of the library of Nineveh, describe a core of herbal remedies of about 200 plants.

560~480 B.C.
Susruta-Samhita, the oldest medical text of India, was compiled.

Melissa officinalis

still used as an incense in Catholic churches today. Onycha is a rockrose that exudes a gum, later mentioned as medicinal by the Greek physician Dioscorides. Galbanum is an aromatic gum-resin that may have had medicinal uses, and some members of the galbanum family are used in cooking today.

The later classical period

Three of the most famous herbalists of all time lived during the first two centuries A.D. Roman scholar Pliny's monumental *Natural History*, written around A.D. 77, dealt with medicinal plants. It abounds in errors but is lively and interesting. Pliny pointed out rather shrewdly that the reason herbal medicine was not better appreciated in educated circles was that it was known best by illiterate herb gatherers, and those who did have knowledge refused to pass it on for fear of losing their source of income.

Dioscorides was born in Greece in A.D. 40 and was probably a doctor in the Roman army. He traveled extensively and prided himself that his knowledge of plants was by direct observation in the field and from diligent inquiry of local sources. The plants in his *Materia Medica* are arranged according to medical usage.

Galen was born in Asia Minor in A.D. 130. He was a renowned physician in his day and became personal physician to the emperor Marcus Aurelius toward the end of his life. He put his considerable reputation behind the writings of Dioscorides, which is probably why they survived into the Middle Ages. Galen was highly critical of doctors who relied on apothecaries and herb collectors for their medicinal plants, and he took pride in his own practical abilities in the field. Ironically, the excellence of his work encouraged later generations to rely on the book learning he so deplored. The term *galenical*, still used today, refers to certain pharmaceutical preparations of plants.

The Middle Ages

After the fall of Rome, classical learning was preserved by monks and nuns in monasteries and the Byzantine Greeks, together with the great Arabic civilization that emerged in the seventh century and swept across North Africa to Spain, bringing with it a golden age of Persian medicine.

500 B.C.
Tzu-I Pên Tshao Ching, the classical pharmacopeia, largely herbal, is thought to have been composed in China.

460-377 B.C.
Hippocrates (right) devoted great attention to diet, clean water, hygiene, and environmental factors in health and disease, as well as the use of plants.

Old Testament Era
Medicinal plants and herbs are mentioned in the Bible. In Genesis 43:11, Jacob commanded his sons to take as an offering "a little balm, and a little honey, spices, and myrrh, nuts and almonds."

A.D. 77
Pliny's *Natural History* was written.

A.D. 100
Greek physician Dioscorides' *Materia Medica* (right) came to fame.

A.D. 130
Galen, physician to Roman emperor Marcus Aurelius, was born.

The Roman Empire
Romans spread their vast knowledge of medicinal plants across Europe. They introduced over 200 important herbs, including rosemary, lavender, fennel, and parsley, into Great Britain.

Rosmarinus officinalis

Lavandula officinalis

Petroselinum crispum

Foeniculum vulgare

The great Persian physician Rhazes (Abú Bahr Mohammad ibn Zakarijá ar-Rázi) lived from about A.D. 865 to 925 and added greatly to the works translated from the Greek. As well as many textbooks on medicine, he wrote vast numbers of prescriptions; for colic he prescribed chamomile, fennel, fenugreek, and the seeds of quince, just as an herbalist might today.

On the other side of Europe in the 10th century, a medical school was established at Salerno, near Naples. Taking the best from Greek learning and Arabian medicine, it flourished for 300 years, and its graduates earned the title *doctor*.

In northern Europe the Anglo-Saxons showed a keen interest in herbalism, and a number of fascinating manuscripts have survived that combine herb lore with magic rather than science. They appear to have borrowed their basis for herbalism from the Physicians of Myddfai—a group of Welsh healers who have been lauded for keeping alive classical medicine at this time.

One of the most famous medieval names in herbalism is St. Hildegarde (1098–1179), the Benedictine abbess of Rupertsberg, near Bingen, Germany. She wrote two medicinal books—*Physica* and *Causae et Curae*—and made the earliest known mention of some north European medicinal plants.

During the middle of the 13th century, Albertus Magnus, a remarkable German botanist and physician, wrote seven books on plants. As a Dominican monk, he was charged with inspecting each of their monasteries. This he did on foot, observing the plants along the way.

At the end of the Middle Ages, the Swiss alchemist and healer Paracelsus wrote many tracts on herbalism. His first interest was in the alpine plants of his native land, but later he recorded the plants used by gypsies and itinerant folk herbalists. Although full of errors, his work signaled the gradual trend away from using whole plants to the single-ingredient medications of the 19th and 20th centuries.

The Renaissance and beyond

The scientific vision of the ancient Greeks was revived in northern Italy during the Renaissance. By the 16th century this had helped give rise to many herbalist-doctors

865–1037

These years saw the growth of Persian medicine, during which two of the greatest Persian physicians, Rhazes (Abú Bahr Mohammad ibn Zakarijá ar-Rázi) and Avicenna (Ibn Sina) further developed knowledge of herbalism.

10th century

The religious Druidic group, the Physicians of Myddfai, kept classical medicine alive by continuing herbal traditions in northern Europe.

1193–1280

Albertus Magnus, a German botanist and physician, increased the European understanding of herbal medicine.

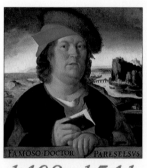

1493–1541

Swiss alchemist and herbalist Paracelsus (above) developed an understanding of single-ingredient herbalism from the folk medicine of gypsies and travelers.

10th century

Medical school established at Salerno, Italy. An adage from the school read, *"Salvia salvatrix, natura conciliatrix,"* meaning "Sage the savior; nature the conciliator."

Salvia officinalis

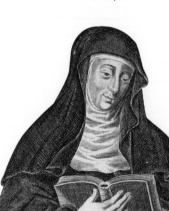

HILDEGARDIS a Virgin Prophetess, Abbess of S.ᵗ Rvperts Nunnerye. She died at Bingen A° Do: 1180 Aged 82 yeares.

1098–1179

St. Hildegarde (above), Benedictine abbess of Rupertsberg, wrote two famous books on herbalism.

all over Europe. During the early part of the 16th century, Leonhart Fuchs (1501–1585) wrote his masterpiece, *De historia stirpium,* which was noted not only for its keen eloquence but also for superb woodcut illustrations. He gave the name *digitalis* to foxglove, and fuchsias were named after him.

Around the same time, a doctor's son called Mathiolus (Pierandrea Mattioli) was singled out by the success of his written works. These started as commentaries on Dioscorides but progressed to superbly illustrated studies of all the plants known to him. It is said that the early editions of his *Commentaries* sold 32,000 copies.

Physicians from Flanders did much to stimulate and develop plant science. The plant genus *Lobelia* was subsequently named in honor of one of them—Lobelius (Mathias de l'Obel, 1538–1616).

The English herbalist John Gerard borrowed (to put it charitably) some of the text and a great many of the woodcuts from continental sources for *The Great Herball* or *Generall Historie of Plantes.*

John Parkinson (1567–1650), herbalist to Charles I, was the first to record some of the more useful medicinal plants native to Great Britain, such as the Welsh poppy and lady's slipper, a beautiful orchid that is now extremely rare there.

Nicholas Culpeper (1616–1654), one of England's most famous herbalists, was severely criticized in his own day for his complete reliance on astrology in his definition and examination of herbs. Two of his books—*Physicall Directory* and *The English Physician*—were enormously popular and have remained so to this day. An important part of Culpeper's appeal was doubtless his genuine compassion for the sick and his dislike of physicians who would rather import an expensive medicine from the East than use equally effective local plants.

BY WORD OF MOUTH

Civilizations in North America, Africa, and Siberia that did not develop a written form of language certainly knew herbal medicine and developed both theory and practice for applications that were passed down from generation to generation. Usually, as was the case in Babylon and ancient Egypt, the function of the doctor was combined with

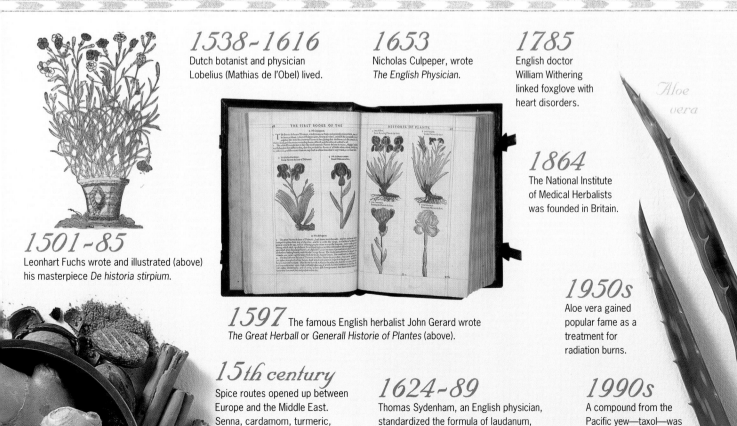

1538–1616
Dutch botanist and physician Lobelius (Mathias de l'Obel) lived.

1653
Nicholas Culpeper, wrote *The English Physician.*

1785
English doctor William Withering linked foxglove with heart disorders.

1864
The National Institute of Medical Herbalists was founded in Britain.

Aloe vera

1501–85
Leonhart Fuchs wrote and illustrated (above) his masterpiece *De historia stirpium.*

1597 The famous English herbalist John Gerard wrote *The Great Herball* or *Generall Historie of Plantes* (above).

15th century
Spice routes opened up between Europe and the Middle East. Senna, cardamom, turmeric, ginger, nutmeg, and cinnamon were introduced into Europe.

1624–89
Thomas Sydenham, an English physician, standardized the formula of laudanum, based on the opium poppy, and modern herbalism began.

1950s
Aloe vera gained popular fame as a treatment for radiation burns.

1990s
A compound from the Pacific yew—taxol—was identified as a useful cancer treatment.

Mint

In biblical times Pharisees collected mint for tithes—taxes paid to the temple. To the taxpayers, mint was considered currency.

During the Plague a posy of such herbs as rosemary, sage, rose, and lavender was used by the rich in an attempt to stave off the smell and spread of disease.

Opium poppies

In the 19th century there were two wars between China and Great Britain when the Chinese tried to ban the import of opium from India into their country.

Today the commercialism of herbs has grown immensely. From medicines and cosmetics to dietary supplements, dyes, and decorations, herbalism has become a huge business.

The Currency of Herbs

Herbs have played such an important part in the growth of so many societies that they have at times been used as currency and come to represent wealth and social position. The importance of the herb and spice trade has led to international unrest and even war.

that of a priest. In Siberia, Lapland, and parts of North America and West Africa, the priest or shaman would induce a state of trance in himself and his patients, sometimes with the aid of hallucinogenic plants, in order to commune with the spirit of the sick person.

The apothecaries and physicians among the European settlers in North America brought their own drugs with them and were at first contemptuous of the idea that they had anything to learn from Native Americans. Fortunately, unlettered people living on the frontier were not so dismissive. Thus it is that European herbalists learned of the benefits of squaw vine, false indigo, blue and black cohosh roots, goldenseal, and many other plants from North America.

FROM CULPEPER TO THE MODERN DAY

The modern approach to herbal remedies may be seen as beginning with Nicholas Culpeper. He advocated the use of natural local flora to cure ills and to help the poor avoid the expensive foreign herbs that many doctors prescribed.

His books brought herbal remedies into many people's homes, and popular opinion forced acceptance of indigenous herbal remedies. This helped to push out the growing numbers of herbal quacks and mountebanks who plied their generally worthless wares around the countryside.

The demand for acceptable herbal remedies that actually worked to combat disease led to greater interest and investment in herbalism and medicine in the 18th and 19th centuries. The growth of patent medicines and scientific testing for active herbal and natural ingredients led to great leaps in the understanding of therapeutic herbal preparations.

Herbalism itself began to branch into diverse disciplines, such as homeopathy, Bach flower remedies, and by the early 20th century, aromatherapy.

During the 20th century improvements in scientific research further exposed the therapeutic powers of plant-based remedies, and the development of better transport and storage meant that the scope for gathering herbs was extended worldwide.

Reassessing herbalism and superstition

There has been a long tradition linking herbal remedies and preparations with magic, witchcraft, and superstition. It is often assumed, however, that if a plant is associated with a superstition, any claimed medicinal use of the plant must be false.

Superstitious fallacies arise when a culture believes in its traditions and practices, even when the belief contradicts personal experience. In the Middle Ages in northern Europe, medical practice was entrenched in superstition, and the majority of people were actively discouraged from using and trusting their own observation. Early civilizations rarely had the luxury of superstitious fallacy, however. Without personal or handed-down experience of poisonous plants, they could easily die if they ceased to trust their senses. Although some herbal remedies may be based purely on superstition, we must not dismiss all herbal remedies as ancient superstitious foolishness.

DOCTRINE OF SIGNATURES

The doctrine of signatures is a view of nature that was popular during medieval times and the Renaissance. It holds that plants created for man's use display a clear sign, or signature, of the organs or illnesses that they are meant to treat. Whether or not nature developed a system of signs as to the medicinal value of plants is open to conjecture. Nevertheless, many coincidences between plant shape and action are borne out by scientific fact. Yellow plants, for example, were thought to be effective for jaundice. Science has since proved that certain plants that yield yellow latex, such as celandine, have powerful effects upon the smooth muscle of the bile duct, taking bile from the liver and relieving jaundice. This doctrine left an enduring imprint on herbal medicine.

STUDIES OF AGE-OLD REMEDIES

Although we have a wealth of historical knowledge about herbs, only in the last century or so have traditional herbal remedies been the subject of serious scientific study.

The 19th century was the great age of patent medicine. Tinctures, cordials, and electuaries—medicinal powders mixed with honey or other sweeteners—were peddled by traveling quacks and also promoted through advertising and at retail pharmacies, which saw a rise at this time. Once plants were shown to have real value, many suffered the fate of becoming known as a panacea. The word literally means "a cure for all things," and many valuable plants bear this optimistic hope among their common names.

Such widespread and unrealistic expectations, however, led inevitably to disappointment and to the steady and eventual decline of herbal remedies, many of which have since been resurrected and scientifically proven to have valid medicinal applications.

Increasingly in recent years, scientific research into herbal medicines has focused on popular traditional remedies. Many clinical studies of the healing properties of some of the medicinal herbs in longest use have shown excellent results. Among the many herbs subjected to clinical study, three of particular interest have emerged: barberry, feverfew, and valerian.

Barberry *(Berberis vulgaris)*
A densely branched shrub with spines and yellow wood, barberry bears bright red berries in autumn. In the Middle Ages barberry root bark was used to treat jaundice, based on the doctrine of signatures, which held that a plant's appearance (in this case, the yellow wood) was a divine sign of the type of ailment it could cure. (In jaundice,

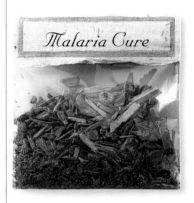

BARBERRY
The ancient Egyptians used barberry as a cure for fevers, preempting the current interest in the plant to relieve malaria, a disease characterized by high fevers.

THE SEARCH FOR A CURE-ALL

Between the late 18th and early 20th centuries there grew a widespread fashion for quacks, unqualified medical practitioners who traveled the countryside selling often worthless concoctions as restoratives and panaceas. This trend led to a growing distrust of herbal and natural cures and may have set back the acceptance of herbal remedies for many years. Fortunately, modern research has brought traditional herbal remedies to the fore again.

MOUNTEBANKS
The market for miracle cures in Europe and North America gave rise to mountebanks—traveling quacks who addressed their audiences from a raised platform or grassy bank.

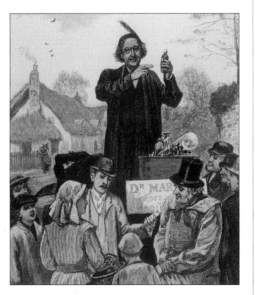

usually caused by liver disease or gallstones, the skin turns yellow.) Investigations in recent years have shown that it may, in fact, stimulate the production of bile in the liver.

The root bark is considered by some herbalists to be an effective remedy for diarrhea, especially when caused by a bacterium. And berberine, a major constituent of the root bark, is used in eye preparations.

The ripe fruit, rich in vitamin C, is sometimes made into jelly; it can be effective in treating constipation, lack of appetite, and diseases of the urinary tract.

The most recent pharmaceutical interest in barberry has focused on its action against disease-causing protozoa. These are microscopic organisms that are carried in the blood of insects such as mosquitos and cause diseases like malaria.

It has also been scientifically demonstrated that barberry is toxic to the causative organism in leishmaniasis, a tropical skin disease that is notoriously resistant to conventional medical treatment and therefore in desperate need of another form of cure.

Feverfew (Tanacetum parthenium)

A bitter herb, feverfew has a strong smell like that of camphor. The earliest recorded medicinal use of feverfew leaves was in Greece, where it was recommended as a remedy for the various disorders to which young women are susceptible. This may be the reason it was so highly favored by herbalists during the Renaissance, as a treatment for painful menstruation.

Nicolas Culpeper in 1652 recommended feverfew to strengthen the womb and allay "all pains in the head." Since the 1970s scientific and clinical studies have shown that feverfew's folk reputation as a treatment for headaches, especially migraine, is well justified. Taking capsules, tablets, or tea daily can prevent migraines from recurring and reduce their severity when they do occur.

In recent years scientists have been studying feverfew as a treatment for arthritis. Researchers have examined the effect that extracts of feverfew have upon the activity

of blood platelets and upon certain changes in membranes. These changes, which are probably involved in the onset of migraine, may also be related to the development of arthritis. So far, however, feverfew has shown little effect when taken internally, but the essential oil is mildly anti-inflammatory when applied topically.

Feverfew can cause contact dermatitis in susceptible individuals. Eating fresh young leaves, the traditional method of taking the herb, caused mouth ulcers in some 11 percent of patients who took part in a clinical trial; digestive disturbances were reported by another 6.5 percent. Nonetheless, even with possible allergic reactions, the outlook for feverfew as a useful herb is very positive. Herbalists today also recommend it for indigestion, diarrhea, menstrual cramps, and delayed menstruation. In France it is used as a mild sedative for combating insomnia.

Valerian (Valeriana officinalis)

The first mention of valerian as medicine seems to have come from the plant list of Isaac Judaeus, physician to the rulers of Qairawan, part of the great Islamic culture of North Africa in the nineth century. In the later Middle Ages it came to be valued as a panacea both north and south of the Alps.

The botanist Fabio Colonna, born in Naples in 1567, tried to overcome his epilepsy with plant medicines and, following the advice of the first-century physician Dioscorides, claimed he was cured by valerian. Other species of valerian have similar reputations; marsh valerian was used by the Menomini peoples of Central America, and there is a valerian mentioned in the Indian pharmacopoeia as well.

Valerian root is an effective calming and relaxing remedy, especially for people who suffer from anxiety, restlessness, or stress-related insomnia. Its action is gentle and it is not addictive, as are commercial sleeping pills and tranquilizers. However, it can interract with other sedatives and should not be combined with them. Pregnant and nursing women should avoid valerian.

A great deal of research has been conducted into the pharmacology of valerian's constituents. The findings tend to confirm the view that a complex interaction of active substances, rather than a single compound, is responsible for the effects and that the whole plant is needed to achieve them.

Feverfew and Valerian Tea
to relieve headaches

2 tbsp chopped dried valerian root
2 tbsp dried feverfew
2 tbsp dried chamomile flowers

■ Mix the three herbs together until evenly distributed.
■ To make the tea, steep 1 tsp of the mixture in a cup of boiling water for 5 minutes.
■ Drink up to three times a day for no more than two to three weeks without a break.
■ Store the herbs in an airtight container.

HERBS AND PHARMACEUTICALS

Although many drugs are based on extracts from plants, there are significant differences in the way herbalists and pharmacists view their medicinal applications.

The first half of the 19th century saw breakthroughs in the study of medicinal plants. Quinine, for instance, was extracted from the bark of the South American cinchona tree in 1820 by the French pharmacists Jean-Baptiste Caventou and Pierre-Joseph Pelletier, who also discovered caffeine in coffee. Quinine remained the principal treatment for malaria until quite recently. Just 15 years earlier in Germany, the apothecary Freidrich Sertürner had isolated morphine from the opium poppy. Opium was at that time probably the most widely used painkiller, but its addictive nature was not fully appreciated.

Some other active plant elements found in the early 1800s are still prescribed today as individual drugs—digoxin, for example, for its stimulating effect upon a failing heart; atropine for its antispasmodic effect upon smooth muscles in the eye, salivary glands,

and bowel; and colchicine for the treatment of acute episodes of gout. Others, like strychnine, were not developed because they proved too toxic for general use.

In North America, Samuel Thomson (1769–1843) developed herbal medicines based on traditional Native American herbs. His simplistic approach to the value of these herbs, however, was dismissed by an American doctor, Wooster Beech, in the 1930s. Beech looked closely at Thomson's herbal remedies and conventional treatments and then combined them to utilize the best of both. This led to greater acceptance of herbal remedies by conventional doctors.

As research progressed, the modern pharmaceutical industry was born. From the outset, herbs and their constituents were recognized as having important healing properties, and yet a major divide arose between

continued on page 30

Pharmacognosy

The term *pharmacognosy* was coined by a chemist in 1815. Unlike pharmacology, which is the study of the actions and uses of drugs, pharmacognosy—literally meaning "to acquire knowledge of drugs"—refers to the scientific analysis and identification of medicinal plants. The rise of pharmaceutical chemistry in the 19th century, along with developments in botanical science, led scientists to examine plant medicines in a systematic way. The isolation of chemical substances from plants showed that there was more to plant matter than earlier supposed. It became clear that there is enormous variation in the substances produced by different parts of a plant, as well as by different plants.

MALARIA

Carried and spread by the bite of a mosquito, malaria is a serious disease caused by any of four strains of *Plasmodium* protozoans (parasites) that infect the blood. The severity and frequency of attacks vary, depending on the strain of *Plasmodium* that has invaded.

The typical symptoms of malaria—recurrent cycles of severe headache, chills, and fever—appear when the infected blood cells rupture and release more protozoans into the bloodstream. Some herbs are toxic to the malaria-causing protozoans and can therefore relieve the illness.

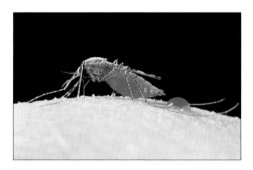

ANOPHELES MOSQUITO
The female mosquito injects malarial protozoans into the bloodstream as she feeds. There are four types of these parasites that can cause malaria in humans.

The Pharmacognosist

Pharmacognosy is a branch of pharmacy that is concerned with the use of plants for medicinal purposes, and pharmacognosists today have an increasing role to play in identifying the constituents of plants that may be useful in treating illnesses.

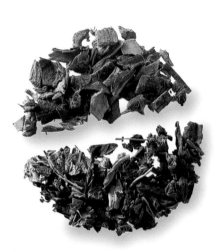

ASPIRIN AND SALICIN
The salicin found in willow and meadowsweet, above, was the forerunner of modern aspirin. Research into salicin's analgesic action led to vast improvements in modern pharmaceutical pain relievers.

Beginning in the 1940s the growing dominance of chemical medicine and the routine use of antibiotics in conventional medical treatment led to less and less use of pharmacognosy in the pharmaceutical industry, and its place in university studies for pharmacy declined. This trend is now reversing, with the increasing interest in herbs as medicine. Once again schools of pharmacy are offering elective courses in pharmacognosy, and more undergraduates are electing to specialize in the subject at graduate school.

What qualifications do pharmacognosists need and where do they train?
A pharmacognosist has a degree in pharmacy—a five-year course in most universities—with a specialty in the subject of pharmacognosy. Botany, biology, and neutraceuticals are major focuses of their studies.

Where do they work?
Pharmacognosists are qualified to dispense medicines at pharmacies, but until recently many worked primarily in the schools of pharmacy that continued to teach their subject. As interest in herbs increases, the skills of the pharmacognosist are in greater demand by the food industry, the U.S. Food and Drug Administration, university research facilities (especially in the area of ethnobotany, or plant lore), and drug companies.

Because plant products per se cannot be patented, drug companies do not seek to use plants directly but try to find and patent unique ways to use plant constituents. Developing, testing, and proving the safety of useful drugs, whether from plants or the test tube, is a long and costly process. But the process with plants does pay sometimes because many plant derivatives cannot be duplicated. For example, colchicine, derived from autumn crocus, or meadow saffron, is used to treat gout, and no synthetic equivalent has yet been found.

There is increasing interest these days in studying the medicinal uses of plants from the rain forests of South America. These may become some of the super drugs of the future.

THE JODRELL LABORATORY AT KEW

The original Jodrell Laboratory at The Royal Botanic Gardens, Kew, in London was established in 1876 to study and analyze the famous collection of flora collected by the the botanical garden staff. This original building, with only four rooms allotted to research, was in use until 1965, when it was demolished to make way for a newer, larger laboratory.

The current laboratory is nearly 10 times the size of its predecessor and has room for 60 staff members. Current work is helping to increase knowledge of seed conservation and of natural medicines from plants, and includes projects like improving fuel woods for the developing world. The laboratory focuses on research, conservation, and furthering scientific and medical knowledge about plants from all over the world.

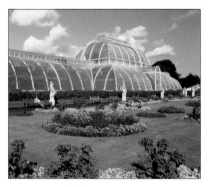

KEW GARDENS
The beautiful gardens at Kew are home to a vast collection of herbs and other plants from around the world. They make an ideal setting for one of the foremost centers for pharmacognosy in the world.

Do pharmacognosists treat the public with medicinal plants?

No. Although pharmacognosists possess an enormous amount of knowledge about plants, their work is primarily in research and teaching rather than in practicing medicine. Some dispensing pharmacists, depending on where they were trained, have a grounding in pharmacognosy, especially in France, Germany, and southeastern Europe, where herbs are commonly sold over the counter, but that is not their primary function.

Pharmacognosy is concerned with the herb at every stage—from collecting, drying, storing, and shipping of plant parts to the processing extracting, and analyzing of their constituents—but not with the consumer. Some exporters and importers of crude plants for drugs employ a full-time pharmacognosist as part of their quality control.

If a complaint is made about a plant product, a sample may be sent to a pharmacognosist for analysis. If you wanted to authenticate a sample of an herbal drug, you could send it to a school of pharmacy that had a pharmacognosy department.

How are herbs analyzed?

The first part of the analysis requires a deep understanding of plant morphology—the details of plant shapes and structures. Through testing, by eye, smell, and taste and then with a microscope, the content of the material can be clearly established. The next stage is to discover whether the material has been mixed with some other inert plant matter or with any nonplant substance, through carelessness or by accident or deliberate design.

PRACTICAL PHARMACOGNOSY
A pharmacognosist must unearth the secrets of a plant at its most fundamental levels. To understand a plant's make-up, a pharmacognosist will dissect and distill the plant until its constituents are distinguishable from one another.

After completing a biological analysis of a plant, a pharmacognosist may be asked to analyze its chemistry to establish if the desired active constituents are actually present in the required amounts and have not been lost through poor harvesting or drying. Chemical tests will also determine if there is adulteration with inorganic fillers and whether the herb is free from toxic materials such as heavy metals.

What are the tools of the trade?

Apart from the skills and "nose" of all detectives, the pharmacognosist depends primarily upon the microscope for authentication of plant material. For chemical analysis, however, plant constituents are first extracted by the application of a series of chemical solvents, then

separated by well established laboratory techniques such as fractional distillation and crystallization.

In recent times the instrumentation and technique known as chromatography has allowed pharmacognosists not only to identify minute amounts of organic molecules that before would have remained undetected but also to separate complex mixtures with a subtlety previously unimaginable. To clarify the structures of natural compounds, the professional also relies on the special equipment and techniques of the analytical chemist. Indeed, many tools and methods of elucidation, such as spectroscopy, X-ray crystallography, and magnetic resonance, are now commonplace technical tools in most branches of science, from astronomy to medicine.

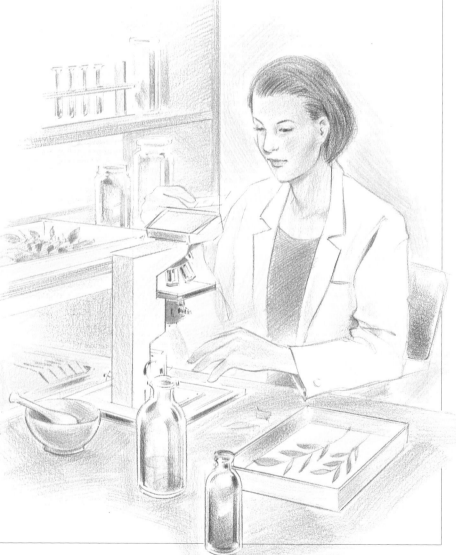

NATURAL HEALING

There is a long healing tradition involving natural products, such as molds, spider webs, lichens, and mosses, to treat wounds and speed healing. They are usually applied directly to the skin, and their effectiveness probably comes from their natural antibiotic properties.

SPHAGNUM MOSS
Toward the end of the First World War, when the demand for cotton bandages could not be met, the British military used tons of sphagnum moss as surgical dressings placed directly on wounds. Fortunately, this folk remedy has not faded from memory and is still used in rural areas.

the pharmaceutical industry and herbalists. Today that divide is narrowing as the medicinal properties of herbs are being explored more thoroughly in the laboratory.

Why doctors prefer drugs and herbalists prefer herbs

The ability to extract single substances from plants enabled chemists to purify and standardize remedial drugs. Doctors work on the basic assumption that if a drug can be shown to produce a physiological effect on a number of people, such as diminishing pain or altering heartbeat, muscle tone, or mood, then it will have more or less the same effect on all people. Of course, individual adjustments of dosage can be made, but on the whole the drug is not tailored for the individual but for the condition.

Herbalists, believing that there is no such thing as a standard patient, place the emphasis of their treatment on the individual. They provide herbal preparations by matching plant qualities with a patient and making minute adjustments in dosage. Only rarely will two patients receive exactly the same treatment for the same ailment.

While doctors generally prescribe a very precise dosage of a single powerful substance, herbalists work with a plant that may contain several hundred different substances. In addition to active constituents that have a definite and repeatable action on the body (as drugs do), the material may contain large amounts of relatively inert material, such as gums, mucilages, chlorophyll, or fiber. Some of this material may have a ballast effect and alter the rate of absorption of the active ingredients. These substances may also influence distribution to the tissues and the action there, sometimes holding back an intense effect or amplifying an otherwise weak effect. Indeed, many of an herb's "impurities" may in fact promote its therapeutic benefits.

Is one person's heartburn the same as another's?

If a patient suffers from heartburn and the doctor considers that the patient is secreting too much stomach acid and not enough protective mucus, a drug that helps protect the

stomach and is also antacid may be prescribed. As soon as use of the drug is discontinued, however, it is common for the condition to recur. If the same patient consults an herbalist, the idea behind the treatment might not seem that different. Plants that modify gastric secretion may be given along with others to protect the stomach lining. However, the object behind the treatment will be to resolve the condition so it does not recur.

Herbalists consider that the complexity of a plant's constituents have a much broader action than that of a drug, and it is not necessary to suppress stomach acid, which is there for the purpose of properly digesting food. Apart from the relative merits of one treatment over another, an herbalist also devotes considerable attention to dietary and lifestyle influences and may recommend some changes, as well as auxiliary treatments such as massage or relaxation exercises.

Despite the contrast between these two approaches, a good number of herbal extracts have been standardized for a particular constituent and are sold in pharmacies, health food stores, and in some regions, herbal stores. In Germany, France, Italy, and parts of Eastern Europe, doctors frequently prescribe such herbal preparations. The popularity of their use is ascribed to their low toxicity and the low incidence of unwanted side effects.

Germany currently boasts the world's largest market for herbal remedies. Figures for 1995 reveal that standardized extracts of *Ginkgo biloba* and *Hypericum perforatum* (St. John's wort) outsold conventional drug equivalents. Recent research has shown that hypericum is at least as effective in the treatment of depression as many drug therapies, without the troubling side effects.

CHAPTER 2

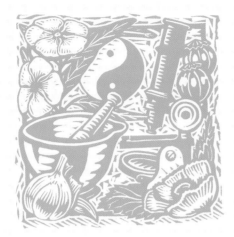

CURRENT USES OF HERBS

---

*Cultures around the world make use
of plants to heal and relieve illness. Familiar
therapies in the West that employ herbal
remedies include Bach flower, homeopathy,
and aromatherapy. Some more exotic herbal
treatments come from as far afield as
Tibet, Pakistan, and Africa.*

HERBS IN VARIOUS THERAPIES

Everywhere in the world there is some form of medicine involving plants. Practices vary from purely folk or home use to sanctioned countrywide systems of herbal medicine.

NATURAL MEDICINE AROUND THE WORLD Knowledge of botanical medicine has developed in every country of the world. Modern herbalism in the West makes use of many healing remedies from different cultures, and one of the major challenges facing medical herbalists today is to keep traditional remedies alive while furthering accurate scientific research.

There are clearly defined differences from one region to another in approaches to herbal medicine. Western herbalism—which originated in ancient Egypt, Mesopotamia, Persia, and Greece—lost favor for some time but was revived during the Renaissance. Today it is widely practiced in Europe, Australia, and New Zealand and is also popular in the United States and Canada.

Chinese herbalism has an unbroken tradition that stretches back to ancient times. It has become renowned around the world and is now practiced in many countries beyond its homeland. Other approaches are prevalent in different parts of the world. These are less well known in the West but are gaining recognition. Despite fundamen-

tal differences that separate various systems of herbal medicine from one another, there are similarities in therapeutic approaches.

HERBS IN THE WESTERN WORLD
The use of medicinal plants declined in the West for decades as the popularity of synthetic drugs grew. But increasing numbers of people are now turning to natural remedies and a more holistic approach to health.

Western herbalism
Herbalists who train in western Europe receive a scientific education that applies the principles of modern biology to medicinal plants, as well as the health of patients. Many traditional folk remedies that have proven healing properties retain a place there.

North American Indian shamans have contributed many remedies to the modern world.

European herbalism is one of the fastest growing in the world.

China's long-lived and complex system of herbal medicine has found worldwide popularity.

African medicine men use many traditional herbal remedies.

Indian Ayurvedic medicine boasts an ancient tradition of herbal healing.

South American healers use the vast resources of the rain forests in their herbalism.

Australian indigenous plants are opening new doors in medical herbalism.

Mainstream medicine in many Western countries has for a long time been unwilling to accept the numerous claims of herbalism, despite the growing interest by the general public. One exception is Germany, where doctors prescribe herbal remedies and there is a growing belief that the natural healing properties of herbs may, in some cases, be more therapeutic than conventional drug treatment. An herbal regulatory group known as Commission E has assessed some 300 plants and identified uses for which they have been found reasonably effective.

Interest in herbal medicine is growing in the United States. There is an indication of movement toward the mainstream in the recent publication of the *PDR (Physician's Desk Reference) for Herbal Medicines,* which is based on the findings of Germany's Commission E. There are also growing numbers of doctors of oriental medicine (O.M.D.), doctors of naturopathy (N.D.), both of whom are trained in herbal medicine, and doctors of herbalism (D.H.)

In Canada herbalists, also called phytotherapists, are not regulated, and so there are no educational standards for practitioners, but some herbal associations set standards for membership. Anyone seeking a qualified herbalist can contact the Calgary-based Canadian Association of Herbal Practitioners.

One problem with herbal remedies is that they remain outside governmental regulation in most countries. This may make doctors and prospective patients less confident in them. In Australia officials have reacted to this problem by setting up a new area of regulation that deals purely with herbs in their own right. In Canada an herbal remedy sold for medicinal used must have a Drug Identification (DIN) or General Purpose (GP) classification.

Aromatherapy

Aromatherapy is a form of alternative medicine that depends entirely upon plants but does not use whole plant tissue, only the volatile, or essential, oils extracted from it. It is based partly on the idea that scents can heal both physical and emotional conditions, and partly on the effects that essential oils have when absorbed through the skin.

In the United States the National Association of Holistic Aromatherapy in Boulder, Colorado, has a newsletter and directories of aromatherapy schools and practitioners.

USING ESSENTIAL OILS SAFELY

Essential oils are highly concentrated and must be used with caution. If in doubt, consult a qualified professional before using them.

▶ Basil, clove, cinnamon, fennel, hyssop, marjoram, myrrh, peppermint, rosemary, sage, and thyme oils should be avoided altogether during pregnancy because they have stimulating and emmenagogue properties that could induce a miscarriage. All other essential oils should be used in half doses during this time.

▶ Essential oils for use in massage should be blended with a carrier oil such as grapeseed or almond oil. To calculate the maximum amount of essential oil you can use, divide the amount of carrier oil—in millileters—by two. For instance, to 60 millileters (1/4 cup) of carrier oil you can add up to 30 drops of essential oil. Never exceed this maximum amount.

▶ Lavender and tea tree oils are safe for use in their undiluted states but should be used only in small amounts.

▶ Do not any use oil other than lavender or tea tree in its undiluted state.

▶ Avoid getting essential oils in your eyes; they can cause permanent damage. Keep your eyes closed during inhalations.

▶ Never leave children unattended with essential oils.

▶ Never take essential oils internally.

▶ Never use more than 10 drops of essential oil in bath water.

▶ Never use a dilution of essential oils stronger than 2.5 percent in a bath.

Homeopathy

Practitioners of homeopathy believe in two important principles. The first is summed up in the phrase "like cures like." This means that a substance that causes the symptoms of a particular illness in a healthy person can be administered to cure a patient suffering from that illness. The second is *continued on page 36*

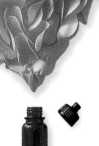

ESSENTIAL OILS
Essential oils extracted from petals are many times more expensive than those taken from other plant parts because petals yield very little natural oil. Rose oil, which cannot be synthetically reproduced, is one of the most expensive; rose petals yield only 0.02% of their oil through steam distillation, and it takes 100 kg (240 lb) of rose petals to extract just 50 g (1¾ oz)of the essential oil. Extraction by solvent, rather than steam, yields more oil, but of a lower quality.

The Aromatherapist

Aromatherapy is the use of concentrated oils from plants to relax muscles, stimulate vital energy, reduce anxiety, and relieve the pain or other symptoms of various ailments. It can enhance both mental and physical well-being.

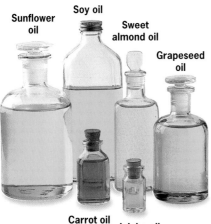

Sunflower oil

Soy oil

Sweet almond oil

Grapeseed oil

Carrot oil   Jojoba oil

OILS AND CARRIER OILS
Before being applied to skin, essential oils must be combined with a base, or carrier, oil. Soy, sunflower, grapeseed, and sweet almond oils make good carrier oils for whole-body massage. For use on the face, especially for people who have sensitive skin, carrot and jojoba oils are more suitable, although they are also more expensive.

Aromatherapy is gaining widespread acceptance in North America for its therapeutic effects. Individuals are trying it to relieve specific problems, and some hospitals have introduced aromatherapy for the benefit of their patients. It's been found that many people recover faster from surgery or illness after aromatherapy sessions.

What training is involved in aromatherapy?
For the interested amateur, intensive courses are available that last one or two weekends or one night a week for several weeks. Such courses may

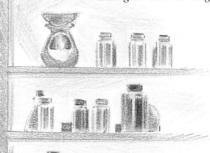

AROMATHERAPY MASSAGE
An aromatherapist who gives massage will tailor your treatment to your overall health and any specific disorders. Most treatments consist of whole-body massage lasting an hour or longer.

be found at adult education centers and colleges. For those who wish to practice professionally, there are certification courses that last from six months to a year. Training generally includes supervised practice as well as classroom time and home study.

Aromatherapists are not regulated in North America, but professional associations set standards and provide information on accredited training programs and practitioners. In the United States you can contact the National Association for Holistic Aromatherapy in Boulder, Colorado. In Canada there are two organizations—the Canadian Federation of Aromatherapists (CFA) in Scarborough, Ontario, and the Canadaian Society of Professional Aromatherapists in Hamilton, Ontario.

In most countries aromatherapy is not seen as a medical treatment and is not covered by insurance. France is a notable exception. Insurance companies there cover the costs of aromatic oils obtained by prescription.

What is treatment like?
Treatment depends on the nature of the problem and the kind of work the therapist does. Some practitioners sell aromatherapy products and dispense advice on which ones are suitable for certain conditions and how to use them. Many give give full-body and/or facial massages. Typically, an aromatherapist will ask questions about recent health problems, allergies, and emotional states.

If you are having a full-body massage, you will remove your

clothes. Because not every part of the body can be massaged at once, however, those parts that are not being treated will remain covered.

A massage therapist uses essential oils incorporated into a carrier oil. It may be a cooking oil, such as soy or sunflower, or a lighter oil like grapeseed, which leaves the patient feeling less oily. A traditional choice of therapists is almond oil; still others use avocado, hazelnut, or wheat germ.

What effects do aromatic oils have?

Aromas can evoke memories and affect emotions, especially if inhaled when the body and mind are relaxed, but there are differences in preferences. A smell that is pleasant for one person may disturb another.

It is important to distinguish between the effects of perfumes and other pleasing but fleeting smells and the influence of aromatic plant oils. Aromatic oils have an added effect on the body when the patient inhales them or absorbs them through the skin. Aromatherapists believe that absorbed plant oils provoke beneficial hormonal as well as emotional responses. Some proponents say that the oils carry a plant's vital energy, which is transferred to the patient.

How are oils selected?

There are about 40 plant oils in common use currently, chosen from the many hundreds in nature. The oils are usually classified according to their effects on the body—for example, whether they are relaxing, stimulating, or uplifting—and the nature of their aromas, such as woody, herbaceous, or fruity. A therapist chooses an oil according to a patient's emotional and physical state and monitors the person's reactions throughout treatment.

The effect of an oil and its aroma can vary considerably, sometimes depending on the soil in which it was grown and the season during which it was harvested. For instance, some lavenders produce an essence that is almost like citrus, which can be invigorating, while other lavenders

have an aroma that resembles that of pine and have the effect of relaxing and lowering anxiety levels. Any oil made from basil is uplifting, with a warm and spicy scent that includes hints of camphor and fruit, while fennel oil refreshes and stimulates and also emits a warm yet fruity aroma. Aromatherapists have good knowledge of the effects of the oils that they recommend.

Are there any side effects?

It is fairly common for clients to become so relaxed that they fall asleep during treatment. If this happens, it is important that they be allowed adequate time to awaken, to get up slowly, and dress unhurriedly. If a deeply relaxed state has been induced, it may not be safe for the patient to drive or operate machinery until fully awake. But it should be emphasized that the person is not drugged in any way; judgment is often very clear and enhanced.

People with very sensitive skin may develop a slight irritation if the blend of oil is strong, but this will show up immediately, and the amount used can be adjusted by the therapist.

Origins

In the 1920s the French chemist Rene Gattefossé's work with plant oils inspired the French doctor Jean Valnet. Valnet used the oils on wounds during World War II, and his 1964 book, *Aroma-thérapie*, made such treatment popular with the general public.

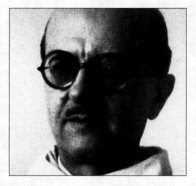

RENE GATTEFOSSÉ
When Gattefossé badly burned his hand in a laboratory accident, he plunged it into a vat of lavender oil. The burn healed so quickly and well that he became intrigued by the healing effects of plant oils.

WHAT YOU CAN DO AT HOME

An essential oil such as lavender added to your bath can enhance its relaxing effects. But remember that oils are concentrated (some are as much as 100 times more concentrated than dried versions of the same plant), and using more than the recommended amount can have the opposite of its intended effect, possibly stimulating and irritating nerves rather than relaxing them. Never exceed the dosage on the bottle.

Added to a basin of steaming water, aromatherapy oils are also effective inhalants for respiratory infections; cinnamon, pine, thyme, and eucalyptus are especially recommended. Care must be taken to count the number of drops used and monitor the exposure time to avoid irritating the mucous membranes.

BATH BENEFITS
Oils should be added to bathwater while the tap is running. Never use more than 10 drops of oil in a bath.

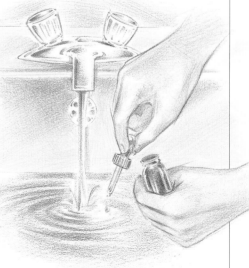

Hypericum is recommended for backache in homeopathy. Although St. John's wort (*Hypericum perforatum*) is also recommended as a back rub in herbalism, the homeopathic remedy is easier to self-administer.

St. John's Wort

Cuttlefish bone

Homeopathy employs fewer herbs than herbalism, but it makes use of minerals and animal substances as well.

Quartz crystal

Sepia from cuttlefish

Herbalism employs many herbs that are toxic or cause side effects. The only substance that may have contraindications in homeopathy is lactose, used in the pills.

Lady's mantle tincture

Lactose pills

Toxic plants used as the basis of some homeopathic remedies are administered in such minute doses that overdosing is extremely rare. In contrast, self-treatment with many plants used in herbalism can be dangerous.

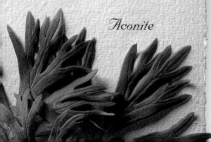

Aconite

Why Use Homeopathy?

Many herbs used in homeopathy are toxic, yet in correct doses, homeopathic pills have no contraindications except for people who are lactose intolerant (lactose is added to pills) and would have to use homeopathic tinctures instead. In general, homeopathic remedies can be safely and easily used over long periods.

that the smaller the dose, the more effective the treatment; if the active ingredient in a remedy is diluted in a special manner (see below), the therapeutic effect becomes more powerful. Because any homeopathic dose is infinitesimal, there is no toxic effect.

More than 2,000 medicinal substances derived from animal, vegetable, and mineral sources are used in homeopathy. If the starting material is an herb, it is used fresh and made into an alcoholic tincture—in effect, a weak herbal medicine. The homeopath makes a series of dilutions, or potentizations, to produce medicines of the required strength. These are most often taken in the form of a white pill, which is placed under the tongue, but may also be granules, a liquid, or an ointment.

Homeopathic treatment is often confused with herbal medicine because so many homeopathic remedies are derived from plants. The distinction, however, lies in the microscopic dosages prescribed in homeopathy and the different approach to treatment. For example, a homeopath may give a minute dose of arnica for emotional shock, while an herbalist would not prescribe it for internal use because it is toxic at strengths required in herbal medicine. Herbalists instead make an ointment of the flower heads of arnica, which can be applied to bruises, sprains, and acne.

Even more remarkable is the case of aconite, a plant so toxic that it should never be put on unbroken skin; some herbalists will not even handle the fresh root unless they are wearing gloves. Yet the homeopathic remedy aconite is sold over the counter for a wide range of symptoms, including sore throat, dry cough, anxiety, restlessness, fear, grief, and insomnia.

The manner in which symptoms arise is considered important by homeopaths. For instance, whether a chill is the result of exposure to dry, cold winds or chilly, damp weather can affect treatment.

Bach flower remedies

Dr. Edward Bach (1886–1936) was an English bacteriologist who became convinced that personality types and emotional states contribute to illness. He believed that the vibrations given off by certain plants directly influence the human spirit. This attunement led him to believe that certain plants were a direct representation of a human emotion. Mimulus, for instance, he saw as the positive response to fear, and so he prescribed it for those in need of courage.

Most Bach flower remedies are made by immersing freshly picked flowers in spring water in a glass container and exposing them to sun for several hours. The flowers are then discarded and the water combined with alcohol, usually brandy. Bach himself discovered 38 remedies. Others have since been identified by other people.

HERBS IN OTHER CULTURES

While herbs have been rediscovered in the West only recently, in other parts of the world they have maintained a central position in the treatment of illness for millennia.

Chinese medicine

Chinese herbal medicine has always had a place in Eastern therapies but is now the focus of increased attention in the West. Chinese medicine has a very firm grounding in ancient beliefs and practices concerning herbs. Indeed, with its long unbroken tradition and huge range of natural flora, China has the largest and most complex repertoire of medicinal herbs in the world.

The main difference between Chinese and Western approaches lies in the philosophy behind treatment. The Chinese believe that everything, both animate and inanimate, has a vital energy that they call *chi*. If the flow of chi through the body is disrupted, the result is illness. Chi can be disrupted by imbalances in the two ruling forces, *yin* and *yang*, and can be returned to its natural flow by treatment with herbs that counter the yin/yang imbalance. Hence, it is not so much the healing properties of an herb that will lead to it being prescribed for a sore throat, but more the yin or yang effect the herb will have on the body's imbalance.

A Chinese herbalist does not simply treat the symptoms of an illness but attempts to restore health to the whole body—a "holistic" approach. Nonetheless, many herbs

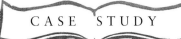

CASE STUDY

An Overstressed Woman

*When both partners in a family work, it is often the woman who bears the brunt
of the domestic load. Juggling the pressures of work, home, and family care can lead to
undesirable stress levels for all involved, and inequality of such pressures may
result in feelings of anger at the unfairness of the situation.*

Miriam is 34 and married, with two children ages 8 and 10. She has worked for the past five years in a supermarket and has recently decided to go to college so that she will have greater earning capacity when the children are older. Her evening classes, which will qualify her for entrance to a university, are going well.

Her husband, Alan, is supportive and helps with the children and housework, but he has a chance for a promotion at work and is putting in longer hours. Miriam is finding it increasingly difficult to juggle her commitments and has started having bouts of nausea and headaches. A friend tells Miriam about the relief she obtained with herbal remedies and suggests visiting an herbalist.

WHAT SHOULD MIRIAM DO?

Miriam and Alan should work out a schedule for sharing home and family duties equitably and delegate a share of the household chores to their children. They also need to set some money aside and prepare a budget so they will be prepared for the time when Miriam is in school full-time and no longer bringing home a paycheck.

If Miriam decides to follow her friend's advice about seeing an herbalist, she will probably be given various herbal teas and bath preparations to help her unwind and relax. These would include valerian and St. John's wort teas to help calm her and improve concentration, and lavender and lemon balm to add to a warm bath for relaxation.

FAMILY
A more even division of family responsibilities can help both partners to feel they have time for their own needs.

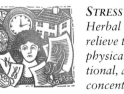

STRESS
Herbal remedies can relieve tension, both physical and emotional, and improve concentration, relaxation, and general well-being.

Action Plan

FAMILY
Decide what household tasks need to be done each week and who will be responsible for them. If unexpected needs arise, eliminate or postpone any nonessential tasks.

STRESS
Consult an herbalist and implement any recommendations within the daily routine.

MONEY
Work out a realistic budget and, if necessary, eliminate some purchases or put them off until later to relieve the pressures of adjusting to a reduced income.

HOW THINGS TURNED OUT FOR MIRIAM

The herbs helped Miriam to relax, and her headaches and nausea disappeared. She had good results on her entrance exams and is looking forward to starting college. Miriam is still under pressure but is strengthened by the support she receives at home. The herbal teas and a daily relaxing bath have also helped her cope. Alan received his promotion, and with greater responsibilities at work, he, too, has found the herbal remedies helpful.

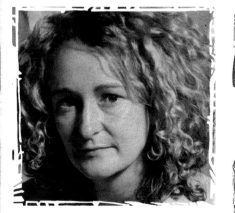

MONEY
Careful budgeting can help relieve the pressure of fluctuations in income.

Herbs and Religion

Herbs have played a major role in most religions throughout the centuries. From classical traditions to African tribal ceremonies, herbs have been used to alter mental states and release the user into a more spiritual awareness. Other herbs are closely linked to deities or used to symbolize them in religious literature and folklore. Some religious groups, such as the Benedictine monks, have made certain herbal preparations their own. The liqueur of the same name is still popular today.

Yage or ayahuasca

South American shamans use a vine called *yage* in Colombia and *ayahuasca* in Ecuador to seek out and heal the soul of a sick person.

In classical mythology a rose is believed to have sprung from the blood of Adonis.

Rose

Benedictine monks adopted the Arab practice of transferring the healing power of herbs into alcohol.

Rosemary in alcohol

Ancient Greek priestesses of Apollo used bay to induce prophetic trances.

Bay

prescribed in Chinese herbalism are familiar to herbalists and patients in the West, even if the theories behind their usage are not.

Tibetan medicine

Traditional medicine in Tibet is essentially humoral, like ancient European herbalism, but differs in having not four but three humors—phlegm, wind, and bile—of which there are no fewer than five kinds of each mixed throughout the body. If any of the 15 varieties of the three humors are put out of balance by the three poisons—desire, hatred, and confusion—the result is either a "hot" or a "cold" disease. Balance can be restored through herbal treatment, using heating herbs for a cold disease and cooling herbs for a hot one.

Ayurveda

This is the name of the traditional medical system of India. Ayurvedic medicine places great emphasis on the temperament and physical constitution of the patient, derived from the bodily humors, or types, known as *vata*, *pitta* and *kapha*.

As in Chinese medicine, medicinal plants are used with very specific, subtle, and complex instructions, and attention is also given to breathing correctly and improving posture, exercise, and diet.

Unani

This healing approach is practiced in Pakistan, where the physician is known as a *hakim*. Unani has some similarities to Ayurveda, such as a concern with understanding the temperament of the sick person and with appropriate diet and lifestyle. Unani was thought to have originated in

ancient Greece and then absorbed influences from Persia, Arabia, and East Africa.

The extent of herbal treatment in the system is astounding. A recent study conducted by the Department of Pharmaceutical Sciences at Nottingham University in the United Kingdom investigated the use of medicinal plants by the Asian community in Great Britain. It found no fewer than 325 species of herbs, some European, currently being prescribed by hakims.

East African medicine

Herbal medicine is offered on a professional basis by medicine men, especially in the Swahili-speaking region of the East African coast. The majority of these medicine men, or *mganga*, as they are called, have been apprenticed by a parent or close relative; others inherit a practice in the form of the *mfuko*, the medicine bag.

As is common in herbal treatment throughout the world, the medicine is personalized to the individual patient. Roots and barks of trees and shrubs collected from the bush are more often used than seeds and leaves; the ingredients are usually boiled together or soaked in water for a long time. Some mganga have also studied the Koran and may therefore also be Islamic teachers, or *mwalimu*. The advantage of these religious and traditional forms of healing, especially for the poor, is that patients accept and feel confidence in the mganga, and this encourages the healing process.

Central and South American medicine

The mountains, lakes, forests, and even the deserts of the Americas in the Southern Hemisphere possess an extraordinarily rich variety of flora that indigenous peoples have developed into a correspondingly rich herbal medicine. In recent decades this system has been threatened because the plants and trees on which it depends are disappearing.

The best-known areas of plant diversity and herbal healing are along the basins of two great rivers—the Amazon and the Orinoco—but a great wealth of plants is also found in the Andes in Bolivia and on the Paraguayan plains. In places like Chiapas in southern Mexico, also in Ecuador and Guatemala, indigenous knowledge has been enhanced with European herbs and ideas, and Mediterranean medicinal herbs, such as anise, are sold alongside native medicines.

HERBAL BEAUTY PRODUCTS

There is a growing demand for products—from skin creams to shampoos—that contain plant extracts to improve their performance, texture, or scent.

Until recently most herbal beauty products contained only a small amount of botanical ingredients, usually not enough to make any difference in their performance. Thanks to a general increased interest in alternative treatments, however, a wider range of good quality botanical products is now available.

The distinction between herbal and non-herbal products is not an easy one to draw because so many contain at least some substance derived from a plant. Even though the fragrance of lemon-scented liquid soap does not come from fresh lemons, the limonene that is used as a scent has its origin in the plant. Dyes and oils from plants have often been added to beauty products to improve texture or color or add a particular scent, but the actual cleansing or skin-enhancing properties have usually been derived from synthetic chemicals.

Products that contain plant extracts or make an appeal to "naturalness" are generally higher in price than chemically based products, but they sell well. This is despite the fact that only a small number of plants, such as evening primrose, jojoba, and witch hazel, are well enough known to the majority of consumers to sell on their own merits. Simply branding a product as "natural" can be enough to give it instant appeal.

SKIN PREPARATIONS

A person's skin type generally falls into one of the categories described in the table below. Dry skin may lack either oil or moisture or both. Normal skin has no extremes of oil or moisture, while sensitive skin is highly reactive to any number of external chemicals, as well as to insects and contact with certain plants. There are four main types of skin preparations, each of which

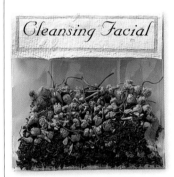

Cleansing Facial

Place 1 tbsp each dried nettle leaves and chamomile flowers in a heatproof bowl and cover with boiling water to make a cleansing facial steam for any skin type. Or use herbs from the table below that suit your skin.

HERBS FOR YOUR SKIN TYPE

Whatever your particular skin type, you can make cleansing, nourishing, and healing cosmetics at home by combining recommended herbs fromdifferent sections of the of the table below in a cream, lotion, or cleanser. For detailed directions on how to make herbal preparations, see pages 75 to 80.

SKIN TYPE	SYMPTOMS	HERBS RECOMMENDED	HOW TO USE
Normal	Fine, smooth texture; no shine or flaking	Lemon verbena, nettle, rose	Cleanse with regular steaming and facial packs.
Oily	Heavy, unrefined texture; shiny surface; large pores; blackheads	Bergamot, cypress, geranium, lavender, lemon, nettle, rosemary	Use fruit or clay masks, exfoliating scrubs, steaming, toning lotions.
Dry	Delicate texture, prone to tightness, flaking, and wrinkles	Comfrey, fennel, jasmine, neroli, lavender, rose, sandalwood	Use cream-based masks and moisturizers, aromatherapy massage with essential oils.
Sensitive	Prone to redness and irritation, especially after using soap or cosmetics	Comfrey, chamomile, lavender, rose	Massage using jojoba oil as a carrier. Always patch test new products.
Combination	Dry around cheeks, neck, and eyes but oily on the "T-zone"—nose, forehead, and chin	Chamomile, orange blossom, nettle, rose	Use rose or orange blossom water cleansers. Massage with a light carrier oil such as jojoba.
Acne prone	Oily, coarse skin; pimples and blackheads	Tea tree essential oil	Apply directly to affected area, 1 or 2 times a day.

can be prepared differently, taking skin types into account, in order to balance or even out extremes of oiliness and dryness.

Cleansers

These remove dirt and makeup and are used in place of soap, which also removes oils from the skin. Cleansers for dry or dehydrated skin have a creamy texture with emollient properties, that is, they are soothing or softening on application. Many are designed to be removed without water.

Herbal extracts used in cleansing compounds for dry skin include cucumber, which has soothing and refreshing juices and a moisturizing effect. Chamomile extract is also soothing and anti-inflammatory. Essential oil of lemon balm has particularly good skin penetration and is added to high-quality cosmetic treatments for oily or acne-prone skin. Orange, lemon, and bilberry extracts are valued for oily skin and for their rich content of alpha-hydroxy acids, which help slough away dead skin.

Toners

Toners are meant to be refreshing and to some extent tighten the skin. Old-fashioned astringent lotions based on aluminium and zinc salts (also used for antiperspirants) have given way to a range of compounds that provide a greater degree of softness to the skin while at the same time toning it. Herbal extracts suitable for use as toners include rose water, which has very soothing properties and is an excellent tonic for sensitive, dry, and mature skin, and sage, which is particularly helpful for toning oily skin because of its astringent qualities.

Moisturizing day creams

These are formulated to hydrate the deeper layers of skin and to provide a protective film over the skin's surface to keep out dirt. A combination of avocado and nettle makes an excellent day cream; the avocado provides vitamin and oil-rich properties, while the nettle has astringent and purifying qualities.

Therapeutic skin preparations

There are many products that utilize the therapeutic effects of certain herbal extracts to repair damaged skin or relieve irritation. Herbalists use comfrey (*Symphytum officinale*), for example, because it contains allantoin, a compound that stimulates tissue regeneration, helps repair damaged connective tissue, and has an anti-wrinkle effect. Allantoin is added to cleansers for its soothing properties and as an aid to retaining the elasticity of the skin.

Cucumber juice is also soothing and refreshing. It has a moisturizing effect that is especially suitable for dry skin types and for first-aid treatment of mild burns. It is one of the most accessible materials for making beauty products at home.

Wheat-germ oil is an excellent source of vitamin E, an antioxidant that protects against environmental damage, and is soothing and nourishing. This oil can also help combat wrinkles and stretch marks.

COSMETICS AND IMAGERY

The packaging techniques used to market herbal products differ little from those for selling other merchandise. In this case, the use of fresh, natural colors and simple typefaces suggests a natural, unspoiled product. Also, the important herbal extract may appear large on the label, even though only tiny amounts may be present. Whenever possible, buy herbal products from established and reputable suppliers or make your own.

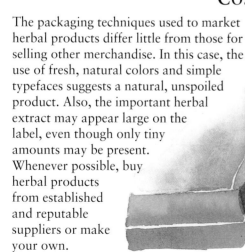

READING LABELS
Ingredient labeling is required on all cosmetics. Except for water, however, most ingredients are synthetic chemicals or plant extracts not familiar to the average person, so ingredient lists may or may not be helpful to the consumer.

Herbal Face Masks

A daily facial-care regimen is essential for keeping your skin both healthy and clean. The occasional application of a face mask will also enhance your complexion.

An herbal face mask, or pack, depending on its composition, may soften, cleanse, tighten or open pores, or stimulate and refresh the skin. It can be tailored to suit any skin type.

The type of masks you use and the frequency with which you use them should be decided on the basis of your skin type, age, and whether you suffer from any skin problems.

Commercially prepared facial masks are often made from wax, gel, or mucilage (frequently containing gelatin, glycerin, and gums from plants). However, they may also be formulated with egg white (albumin) or a milk protein (casein). In some cases they contain special clays or volcanic ash. These are described as argillaceous.

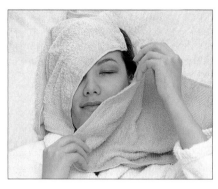

PREPARING YOUR SKIN FOR A MASK
Add 2 drops of essential oil to a basin of hot water and soak two facecloths in it. Cover your face with the cloths and leave them until they are cool.

MASK FOR OILY SKIN

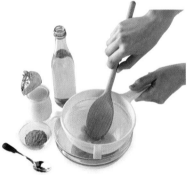

1 *Force the flesh of half a ripe papaya through a strainer into a clean bowl. Stir in 1 tbsp fuller's earth powder and 1 tbsp plain yogurt. Add 1 tbsp orange blossom water and blend to a paste.*

2 *Smooth the mask over your face, avoiding the areas around the eyes and mouth. Leave for about 15 minutes or until almost dry.*

3 *Rub your fingers over your face to flake the mask away, then rinse with warm water. Splash skin with cold water, then pat dry. Store any leftover mixture in the refrigerator and use within a week.*

CREAMY FENNEL MASK FOR DRY SKIN

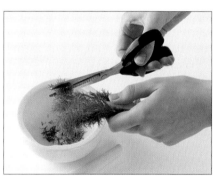

1 *Snip leaves from a bunch of fennel, cutting them into small pieces. Place in a mortar or small bowl and bruise the leaves with a pestle to release the juices.*

2 *Add 4 tsp of sour cream to the bruised fennel leaves and stir together until evenly blended.*

3 *Smooth the mask gently over your face, avoiding the areas round the mouth and eyes. Leave on for about 15 minutes. Rinse your face thoroughly with warm water and pat dry with a soft towel. Finish by applying a soothing herbal moisturizer to the face and neck.*

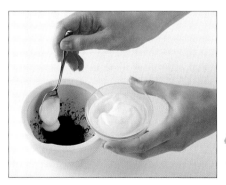

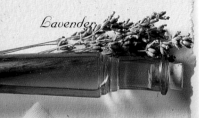

Comfrey infused oil makes a good cleanser for dry skin. Juice pressed from the stalks can be applied topically to relieve painful pimples.

Lavender

Fragrant lavender water is made by infusing lavender flowers in water.

Rose, lavender, and chamomile flowers combined with oatmeal are soothing in a bath. Tie them in a square of cheesecloth and hang the bag from the faucet.

Soapwort is a traditional shampoo base. Make a strong decoction with 1 tbsp of soapwort and rub it into your scalp.

Soapwort

Horsetail contains silicon. To strengthen nails, soak them in a strong decoction of horsetail stems.

Rosemary

Catnip and rosemary infusion can be used as a hair rinse to encourage growth and promote shine.

Catnip

Herbal Cosmetics

It is easy to make effective herbal cosmetics at home for less money than the price of store-bought products. Because homemade cosmetics are preservative-free, most of them should be made with fresh herbs just before use and are not intended to be stored.

Evening primrose oil (*Oenothera biennis*) counteracts the inflammatory effects of the hormone-like substances known as prosta-glandins, which the body manufactures and releases at the site of an injury. Creams containing evening primrose oil can help relieve eczema and irritated skin in general.

The bark and leaves of witch hazel (*Hamamelis virginiana*) produce a powerful astringent that is beneficial for treating various skin conditions. Witch hazel is a common ingredient in many cosmetics, skin lotions, and shaving creams, and sometimes the main ingredient in eye-soothing liquids.

Essential oil of rosemary (*Rosmarinus officinalis*) improves circulation to the skin, which is why fresh rosemary is sometimes used as liniment for stiff, aching limbs. This oil is particularly useful for cleansing oily skins. Similarly, lemon balm (*Melissa officinalis*) has good skin penetration and is sometimes added to high-quality cosmetic treatments for oily or acne-prone skin.

The petals of many flowers are used as healing agents. Those of the cornflower (*Centaurea cyanus*) are incorporated in gentle toners for dry and sensitive skins, while the petals of the red, or field, poppy (*Papaver rhoeas*) have a soothing effect that can reduce the discomfort of many skin disorders. Marigold (*Calendula officinalis*) petals contain oils, healing substances, and active ingredients that cleanse the skin and unclog pores, protecting against infection.

Extracts from the root and leaves of burdock (*Arctium lappa*)—a familiar weed that has clusters of bristly burrs—are believed to inhibit the growth of infectious bacteria on the skin. These extracts can be helpful for oily and acne-prone skin. The leaves and flowers of thyme (*Thymus vulgaris*) are also strongly antiseptic and so help to preserve a skin preparation, as well as protect the skin from infection or yeast growth.

Another therapeutic plant, the horse chestnut, or buckeye (*Aesculus hippocas-tanum*), has astringent properties. It has the ability to reduce the swelling of varicose veins and hemorrhoids and improve circulation, so it is used mainly in strong toners and face masks. In addition, the mildly sedative flowers of this tree may be added to bathwater to aid relaxation, while external compresses made with the seeds or bark may be applied to blemishes and broken blood vessels on the face.

Menthol is a powerful constituent of the essential oils of most species of mint. Very small quantities are often added to skin preparations intended for cooling the skin.

Shampoos and conditioners

A shampoo is a detergent that removes grease, dirt, and skin debris from the hair and scalp without harming the skin or hair shaft. A suitable product will improve the appearance and manageability of hair.

Hair conditioners improve the body and controllability of hair by emulsifying the surface layer and coating it with long-chain polymers and proteins.

A number of plants and their oils have traditionally been associated with a healthy scalp. Rosemary and lavender are well-known examples. Many modern botanical shampoos contain more exotic essential oils, such as ylang-ylang and jojoba. Nettle has traditionally been used as a hair rinse, in particular for treating dandruff, and many herbal shampoos include chlorophyll from nettles for its pleasant smell.

Bath oils

Aromatic essences dissolve well in fixed oils derived from plants, but these cannot be used as bath oils because they form a greasy film on the bathwater and make the skin oily. One solution is to blend relatively large quantities of aromatic oils and emulsifiers with a small quantity of fixed oil.

The label on a bottle of bath oil should indicate that only small amounts are to be added to bathwater, thus allowing for good dispersion. The addition of surfactants also helps this process. These are surface active agents that are crucial ingredients in the production of any emulsion. They work by reducing the surface tension between substances that normally would not blend or stay mixed for long. The addition of surfactants results in a homogeneous product that disperses throughout the bathwater.

THE FUTURE OF PLANTS AS MEDICINES

In the study and practice of herbal medicine, it is crucial not only to understand the constituents and actions of known herbs but also to continue the search for new plants and applications.

While herbal medicines have been used since earliest human existence, it is only in the last 200 years that the development of chemistry has permitted scientists to produce standardized extracts from plants and isolate the active constituents. This process allows greater precision in dosages and eliminates undesirable characteristics such as an unpleasant taste. Modern herbalism even has its own scientific discipline of pharmacognosy (see page 28), yet estimates of the number of medicines currently in use that are derived from plants suggest a drop in the last 20 years, probably due to the increased use of synthetic drugs. This does not mean, however, that herbal medicine is in decline.

Research into phytomedicines, as plant remedies are called, has been accelerating in the last few years. New research has confirmed the efficacy of some established herbal remedies and identified potential new therapeutic uses for others. Some herbs have been studied extensively; garlic is one of them. It has been the subject of nearly 2,500 studies, which collectively have built an impressive picture of its medicinal properties.

THE ROLE OF MODERN DRUG COMPANIES

Following early successes in isolating active compounds in plants, the pharmaceutical industry added a number of highly important plant-based drugs to the pharmacopoeia of modern medicine. There then followed a period of years when drug companies, for economic reasons, focused their attention on synthetic or semisynthetic compounds that could be patented and produced inexpensively after the costly procedure of testing and obtaining approval for them. In 1980 none of the top 250 pharmaceutical companies had research programs that involved plants. Over the past 15 years, however, this picture has changed dramatically, as companies have become interested once again in looking at plant-derived medicinal products. Today over half of the major drug companies are running research programs. So far, this revival of interest has not been matched by research support from funding bodies, with the exception of the National Cancer Institute in the United States, which since 1960 has screened at least 35,000 plants at a preliminary level for antitumor activity—with some success.

THE CANCER CURE WAITING TO BE DISCOVERED

In the past 40 years only three completely new compounds discovered for use in the treatment of cancer have been approved in the West as official drugs. Two of these, the chemicals vincristine and vinblastine, came from the same plant: the Madagascan periwinkle (*Catharanthus roseus*). The third compound, taxol, was isolated from a species of Pacific yew (*Taxus brevifolia*), and researchers had to wait nearly 20 years before it was approved by the Food and

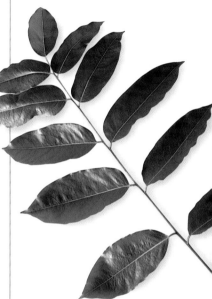

NEW HOPE
More plant extracts are coming to light as remedies for disease. The Australian Moreton Bay chestnut is currently being researched as a cure for AIDS.

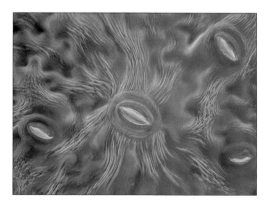

CELLULAR RESEARCH
Electron micrographs, such as this one of an elder leaf, help biologists to study the cellular composition of herbs in order to isolate active ingredients for use in modern medicine.

PRESERVING THE ENVIRONMENT

Given the biological diversity of rain-forest ecosystems throughout the world and their potential to provide important medicines, the rate at which rain forests are being destroyed has caused increasing alarm in recent years. Pressure to expand agriculture is largely responsible for the destruction of areas in the Amazon. Farmers set fire to sections of the forest, then fell the remaining trees and undergrowth with earth-moving equipment. Once clear, the land is given over to pasture, but conservationists warn that such destruction threatens the forest as a whole, through soil degradation and erosion, and the previous biological diversity may never be regenerated.

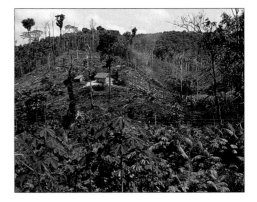

ENDANGERING THE FUTURE?
The rain-forest ecosystem is surprisingly fragile, and the plant, insect, and animal populations that have survived in harmony for millennia are currently under threat from agricultural expansion.

THE MODERN SHAMAN

An area of research that has grown in recent years is ethnobotany, the study of traditional uses of plants and their importance to a society.

In the rain forests of Central and South America, shamans, or healers, often use a mixture of local herbs to cure their patients. Their knowledge of local flora is enormous and could help lead to major breakthroughs in scientific research. Some shamanic herbal remedies are already being studied as potential remedies for diseases such as cancer and AIDS.

Drug Administration (FDA) in the United States. Out of the 35,000 plants screened for antitumor activity, this may not appear to be much of a success rate. When researching cancer-fighting compounds it is important that the efficacy of a new compound is clearly established, that it meets stringent safety requirements, and that its benefits are proven. Add to this the length of time taken to reach approved-drug status, which can include years of testing, and the thousands of synthetic compounds that are also being tested, and the figures fall into perspective.

EXPLORING THE RAIN FORESTS

The extensive rain forests of South and Central America are among the most biodiverse environments on earth; they possess immense medicinal potential. The South American rain forests offer the richest variety of tropical vegetation found anywhere in the world. So far, 25,000 plant species have been identified, but estimates of the number in existence reach more than a million. About one-third of the rain forest flora consists of epiphytes—plants that grow high on the trunks and branches of trees. Since each tree may have its own unique epiphyte species, the potential variety is enormous.

Some of our most powerful modern drugs have come from the few South American plant species investigated so far. Currently official plant-derived drugs are obtained from fewer than 100 plant species.

GENETIC ENGINEERING

In recent years a new area of science—genetics—has come into being. Scientists can now identify genes in both animals and plants that are related to growth, health, and well-being.

In one area of genetic studies, a great deal of effort is being directed at identifying human genes, relating genes to specific disorders, and cloning genes. The hope is that these discoveries will help determine treatments for cancer and other diseases.

The other main branch of genetic research focuses on plant genes. The aim of these studies is to support conservation and further the development of genetically bred food crops in the hope of preventing food shortages in the future.

Designing new medicinal plants

The great majority of genetic research on plants is focused on agricultural and economic needs. Much of the work involves identifying endangered species and building up gene banks—stores of genetic material—that can be used in the future development of stronger, more plentiful crops. Almost invariably the focus is on major economic crops rather than medicinal plants, but our knowledge about the therapeutic effects of foodstuffs themselves expanded enormously in the 1990s through both genetic and other scientific research. It is now recognized that dietary changes can bring about great bene-

Using Herbs for
Natural Pain Relief

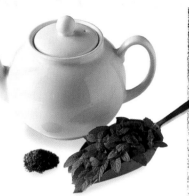

Herbs can be used at home in the form of teas, tablets, or compresses for the treatment of many minor aches and discomforts. If a condition persists or worsens, however, you should always seek qualified medical advice.

The plant world contains some of the most powerful painkillers in existence. One example is the opium poppy, from which all the opiate drugs are made. Many other herbs act gently to reduce inflammation, ease tension, or soothe pain, and these can be used as self-help remedies. Teas can be made from fresh or dried herbs, generally allowing one or 1 heaping teaspoon of dried or 2 teaspoons of fresh herbs to a cup (8 fluid ounces) of boiling water.

Effective painkillers
Aspirin, our most commonly used painkiller, is a synthetic version of a natural chemical found in the bark of willow trees. Tablets containing

extracts of willow (*Salix alba* or *Salix nigra*) may be used to relieve minor pains. Other plants that contain related compounds can also be used, the most common being meadowsweet (aspirin itself was named after an older Latin name for meadowsweet, *Spiraea*). This herb makes a fairly pleasant tea, which can be drunk to ease muscular or joint pains or headache.

Headaches
You can relieve tension headaches with valerian (*Valeriana officinalis*) tea, which is a mild sedative. If your digestion is also affected, mix it with peppermint tea (*Mentha piperita*) to soothe the stomach. Tension and

FRESH AND DRIED HERBS
To make an herbal infusion (tea), you need twice as much fresh herb as dried because a dried herb is more concentrated.

other kinds of headaches can also be eased with catnip (*Nepeta cataria*) tea, which reduces fever as well.

Indigestion
For indigestion due to inflammation of the digestive system, a cup of warm tea made from the flowers of chamomile (*Chamomilla recutita*) can be helpful; for bloating caused by flatulence, try peppermint or ginger tea. All of these herbs are so popular as self-help remedies that ready-made tea bags are available.

MENSTRUAL CRAMPS

Cramping menstrual pains can often be eased by a cup of hot lemon balm (*Melissa officinalis*) tea, which can also settle a painful nervous stomach. Chamomile and peppermint teas, both of which have antispasmodic properties, also help soothe cramps.

Ginger (*Zingiber officinale*), which inhibits the production of prostaglandins (one cause of cramps), is another herb that is recommended for easing menstrual pain. To prepare ginger tea, pour 1 cup boiling water over ¾ teaspoon chopped fresh ginger.

SOOTHING A TOOTHACHE

An acute toothache or pain caused by sensitive teeth can be relieved by topically applying a tincture of myrrh or oil of cloves to the painful area. Although these offer short-term pain relief, it is important to follow up with a dentist as soon as possible to have any underlying problem, such as a cavity or gum infection, diagnosed and treated.

SOOTHING CLOVES
At the first twinge of pain from toothache, take a clean cotton ball or cotton swab, soak it in oil of cloves, and apply it to the affected area. Keep it pressed against the gum until the pain subsides. Pain relief should be almost immediate.

Herbal Myths

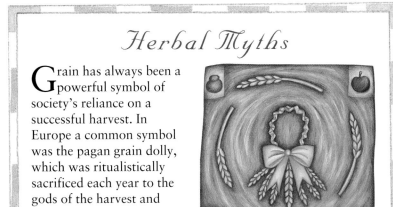

Grain has always been a powerful symbol of society's reliance on a successful harvest. In Europe a common symbol was the pagan grain dolly, which was ritualistically sacrificed each year to the gods of the harvest and later became an accepted figure in the Christian harvest festival.

Research into therapeutic uses of plants has become a worldwide venture, with more and more of the world's scientists searching out the potential of plant remedies.

In the United Kingdom and Germany since the late 1970s, research has led to developments in the use of traditional remedies such as feverfew (*Tanacetum parthenium*) for treating migraines and St. John's wort (*Hypericum perforatum*) for the treatment of depression.

In China a great deal of research has been done on the plant *Artemisia annua*, which contains the compound artemisin. This compound is promising to be the newest and most effective antimalarial drug discovered so far. In India, *Coleus forskolin* is being researched for its potential in the treatment of glaucoma and hypertension.

WILL YOUR DOCTOR PRESCRIBE HERBS?

The answer is that your doctor already prescribes herbs because many conventional drugs are derived from plants. In Germany and a few other countries, doctors prescribe herbal medicines directly, either as standardized extracts—for instance, ginkgo (*Ginkgo biloba*), which is effective for treating vertigo, tinnitus, and age-related memory deficits—or in their whole-plant forms—for example, lemon balm (*Melissa officinalis*) tea, which is useful for easing premenstrual tension—because they are often safer and less expensive than synthetic drugs.

fits in protection against disease, including cancers of the stomach and intestines. Several studies have indicated, for example, that regular consumption of garlic significantly reduces the incidence of gastrointestinal cancer (see page 89) and that eating chili peppers may help protect against stomach cancer (see page 98).

LOOKING TO THE FUTURE, LEARNING FROM THE PAST

The future of herbal medicine lies in combining the best of traditional skills and experience with the careful exploitation of modern developments in scientific research.

The World Health Organization (WHO) has been active for several years in promoting understanding and preservation of traditional, or folk, medicine. It estimates that 80 percent of the world's population currently relies on traditional medicine for primary health care and that the majority of remedies are derived from plants.

WHO also considers practitioners of herbal medicine to be an important part of world health care resources, and as such it is concerned with improving the standards of safety, effectiveness, and quality of herbal treatments. To this end, WHO is involved in promoting national programs of analysis, screening, research, and education.

The current process of screening and testing new treatment applications for known plants or developing new plants now takes place largely in cell lines, using human cells in laboratories for testing the effects of plant substances, rather than in tests on people or animals.

FUTURE MEDICINE

According to geneticists and molecular biologists, the future of drug discovery lies in the ability of scientists to manipulate human genes and develop synthetic drugs custommade for certain diseases. However, this may be a long way off. It seems foolish, therefore, to ignore the plant kingdom as a potential source of new medicines while we wait for the geneticists to realize the potential of their work. Given the huge numbers of plants in the world, there is room for optimism that effective medicines for many diseases will be found through research with botanicals.

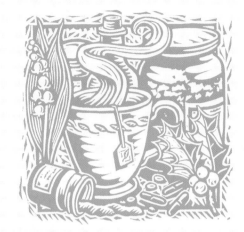

CHAPTER 3

USING HERBS SAFELY

*Over the centuries that herbs have been used
for medicinal purposes, the most highly toxic
plants have been filtered out, leaving only the safer
ones in general use. Herbs like chamomile and mint
have been used regularly by millions of people, with
dangerous side effects very uncommon when they
are taken in proper dosages. Some herbs are less
gentle, however, and must be used with caution.*

FINDING AND PREPARING HERBS

Before using plants medicinally, you should know that your sources of raw material are reliable and fully understand the proper use and dosage of your choices.

The majority of herbs recommended for home use have a gentle action, are considered safe, and are generally suitable for simple remedies or gentle relief from symptoms. If you intend to treat yourself with herbal remedies, there are a few simple precautions you should take to ensure the best results possible. The better you know your symptoms and your herb choices and safe dosages for them, the less likely you will make a mistake.

When you first come across an herb, examine it carefully, noting its color, smell, and appearance. An herb in good condition should retain most of its original color and smell. Compare it to a picture of the living plant. At first you may see little resemblance, but soon you will be able to pick out distinctive features like leaf tips, stalks, stigmas, and stamens, even with dried herbs, which should have most of the detail of the fresh plant. Avoid herbs that appear dusty. They may be old or infested with insects or have been overexposed to light or air.

Treating infestation

Normally, herb suppliers treat them to counteract insect infestation. Most packaged herbs, other than organically grown ones, have been deep-frozen, irradiated, or treated with ethylene oxide, any of which decontaminates them.

WHERE TO BUY HERBS

Buy herbs only from a reputable source. Some are hard to grow, and wild plants can be scarce or inaccessible. These factors raise costs, making it tempting for producers to substitute or adulterate dried or powdered herbs with a cheaper, similar-looking material. Standards for purity require that herbs are not deliberately adulterated, contain a good level of active constituents (to prevent the extraction of valuable essential oils before sale, for example), and that they are in reasonably good condition. However, the monitoring of herbs is very limited in the United States. In Canada any herbal remedy sold for medicinal used must have a DIN or GP classification (see page 50).

QUALITY CONTROL OF HERBS

The regulation of dried herbs or herbs in unlicensed medicines (which have not passed necessary pharmaceutical tests or proved their worth) is less stringent than for licensed medicines. This means that adulteration and contamination from polluted air, soil, or water are not unknown because the monitoring of such products is limited. Medical claims cannot be made, although descriptions such as "refreshing" or "relaxing," and indications as to when it is best to use a product are acceptable in the United States. In Canada manufacturers of herbal products are even more restricted in what claims they make and the language they use.

Most established herbal suppliers and manufacturers maintain high standards and are careful of their reputations because the sale of herbs and herbal extracts is big business today. Better stores deal with reputable suppliers only and are knowledgeable about the products they sell.

Herbs are generally sold in two forms: dried bulk (available in bins, jars, or packages) and standardized extracts (usually tablets or capsules). Dried-bulk herbs are

FREEZING
To kill any insect larvae that may be in your herbs—particularly in roots or flower heads—wrap the herbs in a plastic bag and place them in the freezer for a few days. The frozen larvae will drop off and be caught in the bag. They can then be shaken out and discarded before the herb is used.

THE ANATOMY OF PLANTS

Being aware of the parts of plants used in herbalism and the different preparation that each one requires can help you better understand the method needed for a chosen treatment. If one remedy requires angelica root and another uses saffron stamens, by understanding the structure of plants, you can judge that the saffron remedy will require less preparation than the one with angelica root because stamens are soft, aerial parts, while roots are hard and woody.

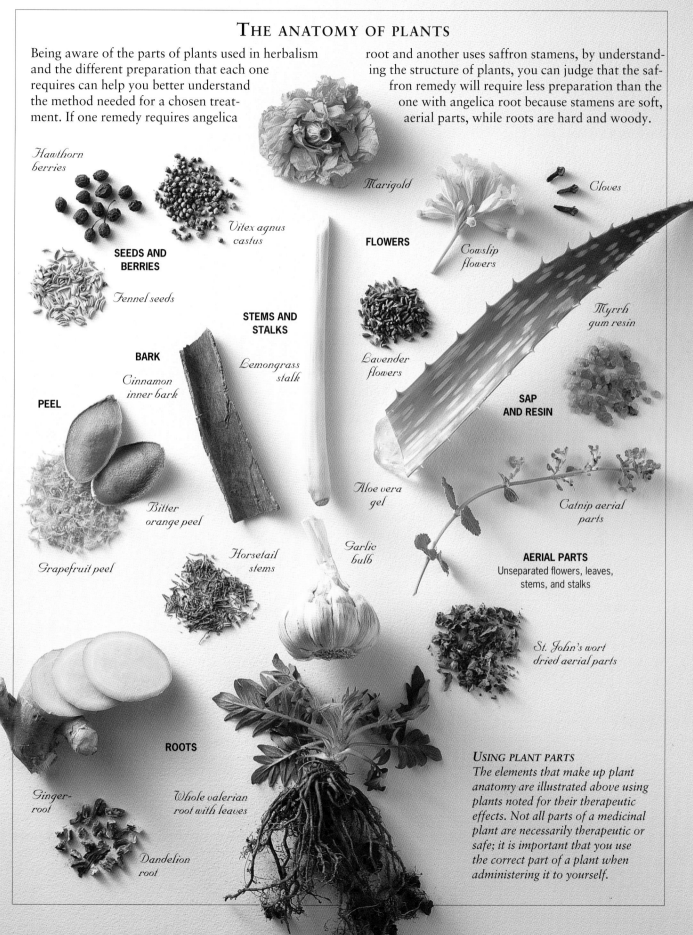

Hawthorn berries

Vitex agnus castus

SEEDS AND BERRIES

Fennel seeds

Marigold

Cloves

FLOWERS

Cowslip flowers

Lavender flowers

Myrrh gum resin

STEMS AND STALKS

Lemongrass stalk

BARK

Cinnamon inner bark

PEEL

Bitter orange peel

SAP AND RESIN

Aloe vera gel

Catnip aerial parts

Grapefruit peel

Horsetail stems

Garlic bulb

AERIAL PARTS
Unseparated flowers, leaves, stems, and stalks

St. John's wort dried aerial parts

ROOTS

Ginger-root

Whole valerian root with leaves

Dandelion root

USING PLANT PARTS
The elements that make up plant anatomy are illustrated above using plants noted for their therapeutic effects. Not all parts of a medicinal plant are necessarily therapeutic or safe; it is important that you use the correct part of a plant when administering it to yourself.

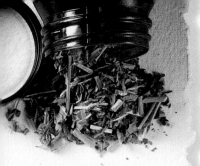

Dark glass jars and bottles are ideal for storing herbs because many lose their efficacy in light.

Correctly stored petals will retain their color and shape; faded, dusty, or disintegrating petals should be discarded.

Brown paper bags can also be used to store dried herbs.

Use several small jars rather than one large one; opening jars frequently can spoil herbs.

Label all herb jars clearly to avoid misapplications.

Storing and Labeling

It is important that herbs and herbal products be treated, stored, and labeled correctly, both by suppliers and by consumers. If these steps have been ignored, you may find that the preparations you have chosen are substandard. They could even be dangerous.

usually safe to use and are generally less expensive than extracts, but the amount of active ingredients they contain will vary. Standardized extracts, on the other hand, have been processed in such a way that the manufacturer can guarantee a minimum level of the principal active ingredients.

REGULATIONS IN DIFFERENT COUNTRIES

Herbs are regulated differently from one country to another. In Germany about 130 herbs are licensed as medicines, with strict standards for composition and purity. A wide range of teas and other herbal products is available, and the licensing procedure for new products using approved herbs is relatively straightforward. The herbal medicine industry competes seriously with major drug companies and supplies a high proportion of prescriptions made by physicians.

In the United States most herbs are sold as food or food supplements rather than medicines. In order to qualify as medicine, an herb must be approved by the Food and Drug Administration as both effective and safe. The cost of providing such proof is prohibitively high and an herb is not patentable. One result is that some powerful herbs are sold with no labeling as to proper medicinal uses or possible side effects, and consumers have misused them. A few herbs that have undergone extensive independent studies do have benefits listed on their labels.

In Canada all herbal remedies are regulated under the Food and Drugs Act. Any herbal product sold for medicinal use must have a Drug Identification Number (DIN) or General Purpose (GP) classification. To qualify for these designations, manufactrers must provide evidence that the products have passed a review of their formulation, labeling, and instructions.

A major problem for legislators is that most herbs are different from foods, food additives, and drugs but are usually put into one of these categories. Canada has dealt

with this situation by creating the Office for Natural Health Products, which will eventually be responsible for regulating herbal remedies, homeopathic preparations, and nutritional supplements. In Australia this problem is being addressed by the Traditional Medicines Evaluation Committee, which includes practitioners of orthodox medicine as well as pharmacists. Thus, while ginseng is classified as a food in North America and an over-the-counter medicine in Germany and Switzerland, in Australia it is a therapeutic substance and is regulated accordingly.

STORING HERBS

Although the medicinal properties of herbs eventually fade, if they have been properly dried and are stored in a cool place, most will keep for up to 12 months or so. Two factors cause herbs to deteriorate. The first is physical—moisture, heat, air, light, and contaminants in the air. To minimize these effects, herbs should be kept in a dry, cool, and dark place. Ideally, the temperature should stay below 15°C (60°F). The second is biological. All sorts of things can attack herbs, including bacteria, fungi, insects, and rodents. In the case of bacteria and fungi, they need moisture to thrive, but the others just need access to the herb. A good solution is to pack herbs in a secure, airtight container like a dark glass jar with a tight-fitting lid. Dry paper in the jar will help absorb any moisture and keep the herbs fresh longer.

You should put a date on your container when you fill it, and refill it only when it is empty. Discard or find another use for herbs over a year old. As a general rule, the fresher the herb, the better it will work medicinally. However, culinary herbs over a year old can still be used to flavor stews, and herbs like lavender or chamomile will make a soothing bath. Lavender or hops can be made into an herb pillow to help you sleep; old hops are actually better than fresh ones for this purpose because the flowers of the female plant, the strobiles, change with age as the constituents oxidize.

HERBAL PREPARATIONS FOR INTERNAL USE

Herbal remedies taken internally are usually in liquid form—infusions, tinctures, decoctions, juices, and syrups—and the herbs need to be carefully prepared to avoid destroying their medicinal properties (see pages 75–80). Each form has advantages and disadvantages. Tinctures are better than infusions and decoctions for extracting the volatile oils from herbs. Tinctures and syrups also preserve herbs better than dry storage, whereas infusions and decoctions will keep in the refrigerator for a couple of days only, and juices for a week or so.

The medicinal substances in plants are generally either water or oil soluble. Water-soluble compounds occur in the fluid inside or outside the plant cell, while oil-soluble compounds are found in special glands, flowers, seeds, or the cell walls and are therefore more difficult to extract. Adding hot water to herbs for infusions and decoctions extracts mainly the water-soluble components, such as glycosides, tannins, and flavonoids. The heat of the liquid does extract some volatile oils also, however, and aromatic herbs like thyme and chamomile should be prepared in a covered container to prevent the oils from evaporating.

Prolonged heat changes the properties of some constituents, so decoctions—made by simmering herbs—should generally be reserved for woody material. Silicates, starch, and mucilage, which are water based, can be extracted only by hours of soaking.

Retaining essential oils

Some herbs, elecampane and lemon balm, for example, lose most of their essential oil even with moderate heat, and a fresh tincture or a syrup made by cold infusion is an excellent way to preserve their properties.

Another way to prepare herbs that are best used fresh is to extract the juice. Fresh plant juices are now becoming quite widely available in many health food and juice stores, but you can also make your own at home with a juice extractor.

HERBAL PREPARATIONS FOR EXTERNAL USE

For external use, herbs may be prepared as poultices or lotions (which are water based), or as infused oils, creams, or ointments (see page 79). Ointments and creams are made up of tiny droplets of oily liquids that are mixed with and dispersed in a watery medium, so they can incorporate both water-soluble and oil-soluble constituents.

Infused oils generally keep very well, but creams need refrigeration and some form of preservative, herbal or otherwise, if they are to last more than a few weeks. Always discard herbal remedies if they are old or show signs of aging or mold.

READING THE SIGNS OF FRESHNESS

Before applying an herbal remedy, check that there are no signs of aging, discoloration, or mold. The life span of all remedies is limited; the length of time it will keep depends on the type (see pages 75–80) and how it is stored. If you have any reason to suspect that your remedy is not in good condition, discard it.

Poultices should be discarded after use. Do not reheat any herbal mixture for a poultice.

CHECK FOR FRESHNESS
There are ways of checking that any herbal preparation is in good condition. Good color and texture and a general lack of damage are useful checks for all.

Compresses should retain their smell and color for two days, but should be discarded thereafter.

Infusions and decoctions should smell fresh and retain their color. Too much sediment may be a sign of age.

Creams and ointments should be free of dry cracks, mold, and discoloration.

Capsules must be dry and the cases undamaged. Discard capsules if there is any sign of damage or discoloration to the cases.

CLASSIFYING HERBS BY USE

When an herb has a therapeutic action, its effect is often described using specific terminology. Understanding these terms can be very useful when selecting herbs.

When choosing an herbal remedy, you want the one that is most suitable to your symptoms and least likely to cause any problems or side effects. Becoming familiar with the terms used to describe the actions of herbs will help you understand their effects and select the best remedy for your condition.

Once you have decided on an herb to relieve your problem, find out what other actions it may have and if there are any cautions or contraindications. It could be that the carminative you've selected to ease your pregnancy-related indigestion is one that should be avoided by pregnant women

HERBS AND DIGESTIVE PROBLEMS
Some of the best-known and most widely used herbal remedies are those that prevent or relieve digestive disorders.

An herb that stimulates gastric juices and other digestive functions is described as having a bitter action. Bitters are taken to stimulate appetite and promote digestion and can help to relieve indigestion as well. Because of their digestive properties, bitter herbs can also help relieve the distress caused by food allergies. Similar to a bitter is an aperitive herb, which can be taken to revive diminished appetite due to a minor, feverish illness or stress. Normal appetite usually returns of its own accord after the underlying condition has been cured, but a gentle aperitive action may help to bring this about more quickly.

Indigestion and colic can be eased with carminative herbs because these help to relieve and expel gas while also calming intestinal spasms and soothing the gut wall. Herbs that generally calm the stomach are

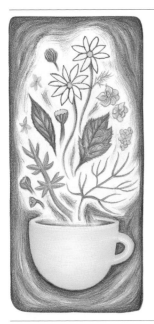

THERAPEUTIC ACTIONS OF HERBS

The chart over the next four pages offers examples of herbs that have particular therapeutic actions, as well as descriptions of those actions. When you have

selected an herb, carefully follow the instructions for preparation and dosage in Chapters 4, 5, and 6 to achieve the maximum benefit from your remedies.

TERM	ACTION	HERB EXAMPLE
Abortifacient	Increases the risk of or causes abortions or miscarriages	Thuja
Adaptogenic	Improves body's adaptability to cope with stress	Ginseng
Alterative	Speeds up or slows down the body's metabolism as needed	Red clover
Analgesic	Relieves pain	Willow bark
Anodyne	Relieves pain	Cloves
Anthelmintic	Destroys and expels intestinal worms	Wormwood
Anticatarrhal	Combats and relieves congestion in the respiratory tract	Marsh mallow
Antiemetic	Suppresses or relieves vomiting and feelings of nausea	Fennel

called stomachics and may be used to relieve many digestive disorders.

For mild constipation an herbalist will recommend aperient herbs to gently stimulate the normal movement of the bowel. Although laxatives are sometimes advised, they encourage an abnormal evacuation of the bowel by irritating the lining of the upper intestine. This causes a reflex action in the digestive tract that stimulates the muscles in the bowel and increases their activity. For a more intensely laxative action to relieve severe constipation, an herbalist will usually recommend a cathartic herb to produce a strong, positive bowel evacuation. Exceptionally laxative herbs that cause copious movement and evacuation of the bowel are called purgatives. These have a violent effect and should be used with extreme caution.

A cholagogue stimulates the liver to produce bile, which is necessary for healthy digestion. Cholagogic herbs are generally recommended to treat liver disease.

Any substance that suppresses or relieves vomiting or feelings of nausea is called an antiemetic. Careful consideration should be given to using antiemetics because vomiting can be the body's way of clearing unwanted or dangerous substances from the stomach.

Anthelmintic and vermicidal herbs are used by herbalists to destroy and expel intestinal worms, while antiprotozoal herbs kill larger infective parasites such as the protozoans that cause malaria.

HERBS FOR UROGENITAL DISORDERS
Urogenital problems such as cystitis or menstrual pain usually respond well to herbal remedies, and there are some herbs that are particularly suited to urogenous complaints. Diuretics, for example, provoke an increase in the flow of urine, either by increasing blood flow to the kidneys or by reducing the amount of water reabsorbed by them. Diuretic herbs provide effective relief from urinary infections.

Herbs that increase the risk of a miscarriage are called abortifacients. These can damage a fetus but will not necessarily terminate a pregnancy, and should never be taken in an attempt to end one. A partial or unsuccessful termination can be very dangerous and distressing. Some abortifacients may have other properties, but they should never be taken by pregnant women to treat other disorders because of the risk involved. The term emmenagogue is sometimes applied to abortifacients because they can induce menstrual discharge.

TERM	ACTION	HERB EXAMPLE
Anti-infective	Prevents infection	Echinacea
Antiprotozoal	Kills larger infective parasites	Cinchona
Antipyretic	Counteracts and reduces fever	Meadowsweet
Antispasmodic	Relieves the intensity of excessive muscle contractions	Cramp bark
Antitussive	Relieves coughing	Wild cherry bark
Aperient	Mildly laxative—stimulates the normal evacuation of the bowel	Dandelion
Aperitive	Revives diminished appetite	Gentian
Astringent	Dries and creates a protective layer on exposed skin and mucous membranes	Tormentil
Bacteriocidal	Attacks and destroys bacteria	Thyme
Bacteriostatic	Inhibits or retards the growth of bacterial infections	Echinacea
Bitter	Stimulates gastric juices and other digestive functions	Wormwood
Carminative	Relieves flatulence, calms intestinal spasms, soothes the gut wall	Fennel

▶ *p. 54*

HERBS AND THE SKIN

Many skin conditions can be effectively treated with herbal remedies. The remedies are usually applied topically in the form of an ointment, cream, or poultice.

Herbs with astringent properties create a protective layer on exposed skin and the mucous membranes, thus protecting against irritation and inflammation.

Emollient herbs soothe the skin and can be used to relieve rashes. They tend to have a gentle action, and few, if any, cause side effects. Rubefacient herbs cause the skin to redden and become warm because they dilate the blood vessels beneath the skin's surface. The increased blood flow improves the cleansing and nourishing of the tissue.

An alterative herb changes the body's metabolism to increase the efficiency of, among other things, elimination of toxins that can lead to skin disease.

Any herbs that promote wound healing are described as vulnerary. They are generally applied topically to the damaged area.

HERBS AND EMOTIONAL HEALTH

Certain herbs are used for the therapeutic effect they have on the nervous system. Some induce relaxation, while others stimulate positive emotions. An adaptogen, for example, helps to maintain a healthy stress response and improves both mental and physical resistance to stress. Adaptogenic herbs are often recommended for stress-related disorders such as insomnia.

Conditions that may stem from nervous tension, such as irritable bowel syndrome and some headaches, may respond well to a relaxant. These herbs reduce muscular and nervous tension without affecting mental alertness in the way that a conventional tranquilizer would.

Sedatives act on the nervous system to reduce nervous activity and, unlike relaxants, may cause drowsiness and dull mental alertness. Herbs that are described as thymoleptic have an antidepressant action and can help to lift mood.

HERBS AND THE BLOOD

Blood pressure and blood sugar problems react well to herbal treatment. Hypertensive herbs, those that raise blood pressure, can be used to improve poor circulation and ease the dizziness and fainting related to low blood pressure. Hypotensive herbs, those that lower blood pressure, can help relieve hypertension and thus reduce the risk of heart disease and stroke. Herbs described as hypoglycemic have the ability to lower blood sugar levels.

Herbs with a vasodilatory action relax and open blood vessels, allowing the blood to flow more freely. These are recommended for conditions such as angina.

Styptic, or hemostatic, herbs act to stop bleeding and other discharges, such as mucus, both internally and externally. This action occurs whether the herbs are applied topically or taken internally.

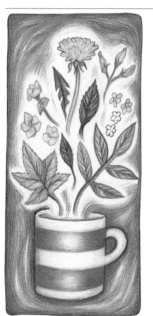

TERM	ACTION	HERB EXAMPLE
Cathartic	Intensely laxative; purges the bowel	Senna
Cholagogic	Stimulates the liver to excrete bile	Goldenseal
Demulcent	Soothes sore or infected membranes	Slippery elm
Diaphoretic	Increases perspiration, helps to reduce a fever	Elder flower
Diuretic	Provokes an increase in the flow of urine	Dandelion leaf
Emmenagogic	Induces menstrual discharge	Mugwort
Emollient	Soothes the skin	Marsh mallow
Expectorant	Stimulates bronchial passages, soothes respiratory tract, relieves bronchial spasm, loosens catarrhal secretions	Mullein
Febrifugal	Reduces a fever	Meadowsweet
Fungicidal	Suppresses and kills fungi	Garlic
Galactagogue	Promotes the flow of milk in nursing mothers	Fennel
Hypertensive	Increases blood pressure	Licorice
Hypoglycemic	Lowers blood sugar	Garlic

HERBS AND RESPIRATION

Inhalants are an obvious choice for treating respiratory disorders because the active constituents can reach the affected area directly. Other preparations can also be very effective. Anticatarrhal herbs, for example, help to combat and relieve congestion in the respiratory tract. When a buildup of phlegm secreted from the mucous membranes blocks the passage of air to the lungs and causes difficulties in breathing, anticatarrhal herbs will help clear the airways.

Antitussive herbs relieve coughing. Most herbal treatments for coughs kill bacteria and loosen and expel mucus.

Disorders of the bronchial passages, such as asthma or a cough caused by excess phlegm, may respond well to expectorant herbs. These either stimulate activity in the bronchial passages, leading to a more productive cough, or soothe the lining of the upper digestive tract, which in turn helps to relieve bronchial spasms and loosen catarrhal excretions.

Any herb described as a demulcent will have a soothing action when applied to sore or infected membranes. Such herbs are often used to relieve coughs and sore throats.

HERBS AND GENERAL PROBLEMS

Many herbs have wide-reaching actions that can be applied to a diverse number of health complaints in different parts of the body. Any herb that acts on a fever, reducing the high temperature, is called a febrifuge. Such herbs either induce sweating in the body, which dries on the skin and lowers the overall temperature of the patient, or they have a directly cooling effect on the system. Diaphoretic herbs also promote sweating and can help to reduce a temperature. Conditions for which fever is one of the symptoms, such as influenza, can be relieved by antipyretic herbs.

Herbs that relieve pain are said to be analgesic, or anodyne. These are sometimes applied externally to the affected area, or they may be taken internally.

Any herb that attacks and destroys bacteria in the body is said to be bacteriocidal (antibacterial is another way of describing it). An herb that inhibits or retards the growth of bacterial infections and prevents bacterial replication is bacteriostatic.

Fungicidal herbs act to suppress and kill fungi, such as those that cause athlete's foot. Botanicals that act to kill viruses, such as the common cold, are known as viricidal, whereas herbs that inhibit and retard the growth of viral infection by preventing replication of a virus, as opposed to killing it, are described as virostatic.

A substance that helps to seal body tissues against infection is known as an anti-infective. Herbs that have anti-infective actions are often applied topically.

Preventing or curing spasmodic convulsions, spasms, or cramps by relieving the intensity of excessive muscle contractions can be achieved with antispasmodic herbs.

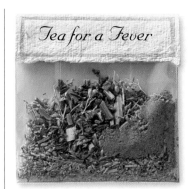

Tea for a Fever

FEBRIFUGAL TEA
A hot infusion made from diaphoretic and febrifugal herbs, such as yarrow, comfrey, and cayenne, will increase perspiration and help to reduce a high fever. Place 1 tsp each of dried yarrow and comfrey in a cup, add a pinch of cayenne, and pour on hot but not boiling water. Sip one cup four times a day.

TERM	ACTION	HERB EXAMPLE
Hypotensive	Lowers blood pressure	Yarrow
Laxative	Promotes the evacuation of the bowel	Rhubarb
Purgative	Causes a copious movement and evacuation of the bowel	Cascara sagrada
Relaxant	Reduces muscular and nervous tension	Cramp bark
Rubefacient	Reddens and warms the skin	Rosemary
Sedative	Reduces nervous activity	Valerian
Stomachic	Comforts the stomach	Lemon balm
Styptic or hemostatic	Stops bleeding and other discharge	Agrimony
Thymoleptic	Lifts mood – antidepressant	St. John's wort
Vasodilatory	Relaxes and opens blood vessels	Chamomile
Vermicidal	Kills intestinal worms	Garlic
Viricidal or virostatic	Kills viruses or retards their growth	Echinacea
Vulnerary	Promotes wound healing	Aloe vera

Dangerous Herbs

Many toxic herbs are now well recognized, and herbalism relies on plants with a good safety record and gentle actions. Accidental poisoning, however, is by no means uncommon.

Dangerous or poisonous plants can often be found growing alongside common edible herbs in parks, the countryside, and gardens. If you are gathering your own herbs, it is imperative that you be absolutely certain of their identities. Some, like foxglove, yield useful medicines but are highly toxic in their natural state. Some, like yew, have enticing yet poisonous berries; others, like fool's parsley, look very similar to edible plants. For these reasons you must be confident of their identification and properties before using them. If you have any doubt about plants you are harvesting, avoid them rather than take a risk.

CORRECT IDENTIFICATION

Before gathering plants, always look up all the identifying characteristics of an unfamiliar herb in a reliable reference book and then cross-reference it with another book to be absolutely sure. Some plants, both edible and poisonous, share the same common name; therefore checking against the scientific, or Latin, name is a more reliable indication of what you are picking.

If you are purchasing a potentially toxic herb for medicinal use, you must follow the herbalist's instructions precisely. If you experience any adverse reactions, stop taking the medication and seek help immediately from a qualified herbalist, doctor, or poison control center. The herbs in this section are known to be toxic and should never be used without professional advice.

POISONOUS HERBS

Some poisonous herbs have very powerful emetic or purgative effects, while others can cause paralysis, extreme sedation, or heart failure. The majority have been used in the past in life-threatening circumstances for which modern drugs—most of which are toxic in high doses—were unavailable or could not be used. Several of the less toxic plants are still used by medical herbalists, who have the training to use them safely.

COMMON CONFUSIONS

Some poisonous herbs are harder to spot than others, and a few are easily confused with common harmless plants, which makes the gathering of them by an inexperienced person all the more dangerous.

Daffodil bulb (*Narcissus pseudo-narcissus*)

The bulb of a daffodil is similar in shape and size to a small onion but is very toxic. These poisonous bulbs, found in gardens and parks, can cause vomiting and paralysis. Although most plant bulbs look a little like onions, none should be eaten because they can all cause gastric upsets or worse.

Fool's parsley (*Aethusa cynapium*)

It is best not to pick any plant in the wild that looks like parsley; many members of its family (the carrot family) are poisonous and very difficult to distinguish from their edible

PAST LESSONS
History is littered with tales of failed cures and accidental fatal doses from toxic plants. There are also many examples of deliberate poisonings and suicides. One such case is that of Thomas Chatterton (shown in the painting below by Henry Wallace). The notorious English forger-poet poisoned himself with arsenic.

cousins (one difference between garden parsley and fool's parsley is that the first has yellowish flowers, while the second has white ones). Although the family includes familiar culinary plants such as celery and cilantro, it is safest to buy these from a reputable nursery or greengrocer.

Despite the poisonous properties of fool's parsley, its juice is used by some herbalists to make poultices and to treat diarrhea and gastroenteric problems.

Arnica (*Arnica Montana*)

Although arnica is used in a very diluted form in homeopathic remedies and is an ingredient in some over-the-counter creams for treating bruises, sprains, and skin irritations, it is a highly poisonous plant. Its external use can produce serious allergic reactions in some people, and if taken internally, arnica can cause a violent stomach upset and cramps, muscular weakness, changes in pulse rate, and death.

POISONOUS HERBS TO AVOID

Many of the dangerous herbs mentioned in the chart below are commonly found in parks and gardens, as well as in the wild. If you have pets or small children, make sure that they don't try to eat any of these plants. If a toxic plant is accidentally ingested, contact the nearest poison control center or EMS immediately.

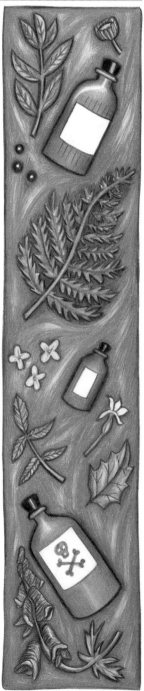

LATIN NAME	COMMON NAMES	POISONOUS PART	EFFECTS	HABITAT
Aconitum napellus	Monkshood, Aconite, Wolfsbane	All parts	Extreme sedation, coma, death	Woods, scrubland, gardens, mountain pastures
Arum maculatum	Lords and ladies	All parts, esp. berries	Severe irritations	Woods, hedgerows
Atropa belladonna	Deadly nightshade	All parts	Delirium, death	Woods, gardens
Chelidonium majus	Celandine	All parts	Nausea, dysentery	Hedges, wasteland
Cicuta virosa	Water hemlock, Cowbane	All parts, especially the root	Convulsions, death	Ditches, marshes
Daphne mezereum	Mezereon, Spurge laurel	All parts	Severe contact irritation	Woods, gardens
Datura stramonium	Thorn apple, Jimsonweed	All parts	Delirium, heart arrhythmias, respiratory failure	Wasteland, barnyards, gardens
Dryopteris filix-mas	Male fern, Bear's paw root	All parts	Paralysis, coma, blindness	Forests, shady banks
Helleborus niger	Black hellebore	All parts, especially the root	Diarrhea, vomiting, heart failure	Woods, scrubland, parks, gardens
Helleborus viridis	Green hellebore	All parts, especially the root	Diarrhea, vomiting, heart failure	Woods, scrubland, parks, gardens
Polygonatum multiflorum	Solomon's seal	Fruits	Nausea, diarrhea	Woods, gardens
Prunus laurocerasus	Cherry laurel	Leaves, fruit	Paralysis, respiratory failure	Parks, gardens
Sedum acre	Wallpepper, Common stonecrop	All parts	Diarrhea, vomiting	Walls, rocky soils
Senecio jacoboea	Ragwort	All parts	Liver disease	Grassland, gardens
Senecio vulgaris	Groundsel	All parts	Liver disease	Grassland, gardens
Tamus communis	Black bryony	All parts	Gastric irritation, vomiting	Roadsides, scrubland
Tanacetum vulgare	Tansy	All parts	Gastric irritation	Wasteland, hedges

COMMON DANGEROUS HERBS

Many highly dangerous herbs can be found in fields, wooded areas, and gardens, by roadsides and rivers, and in parks and vacant lots. Some have pretty flowers and attractive berries; others bear remarkable resemblances to favorite common garden flowers, but almost all, if taken internally, can cause violent reactions and lead to symptoms ranging from vomiting to delirium, palpitations, hallucinations, and even death.

When applied professionally, however, the active properties of these poisonous plants can be used to treat many disorders, from respiratory problems to muscular pain, and they should not be dismissed from the domain of herbal medicine. It is recommended, however, that none of the herbs in this section be harvested or used for self-treatment in any form.

In most instances all parts of the plant are highly poisonous, with some parts having a more violent action than others, and should be used only with professional medical supervision. In the event of accidental poisoning, the patient should receive immediate medical attention in a poison conrol center or emergency room, and the attending physician be told or shown which plant is involved.

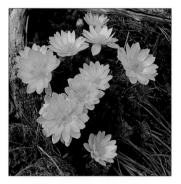

Yellow pheasant's eye

Adonis vernalis YELLOW PHEASANT'S EYE

Also known as adonis, false hellebore, and oxeye, this green-ribbed plant grows in gardens and forests, producing single bright yellow flowers in the spring.

Although all parts of this herb are extremely toxic, it has become favored in professional use as a heart sedative and a treatment for hypertension. It has also been found to contain certain active ingredients similar to those found in foxglove, which can help to increase the efficiency of the heart. Nevertheless, no type of pheasant's eye should ever be gathered for home use or administered as self-treatment.

Poisoning from the plant can lead to diarrhea, vomiting, paralysis, and heart failure. Yellow pheasant's eye is rare and is legally protected in many parts of western Europe.

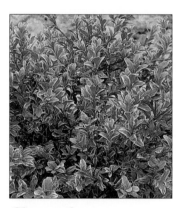

Boxwood

Buxus sempervirens BOXWOOD

A shrub or small evergreen tree, boxwood produces yellow-green flowers in spring and has tough, toxic wood and oblong, glossy, dark green leaves. Boxwood can often be found in parks and gardens as an ornamental plant, particularly in formal designs.

All parts of boxwood are poisonous, but the leaves and seeds are particularly toxic and have been known to cause death in animals that have eaten them.

Boxwood has sedative and narcotic properties. Homeopaths use a tincture made from fresh boxwood leaves to relieve fevers, urinary tract infections, and rheumatism, but the minute quantities used are harmless.

Poisoning from boxwood can lead to severe abdominal pain, vomiting, and diarrhea, often with blood. For herbal treatments, boxwood should be used only under professional guidance.

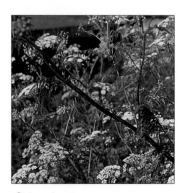

Hemlock

Conium maculatum HEMLOCK

Commonly found in open woods, by roadsides, and often near water, hemlock has an off-putting smell that has been likened to mouse urine. This smell and the purple patches that appear on the stem distinguish hemlock from other members of its family (Umbelliferae), such as parsley. In summer the plant produces clusters of tiny white flowers that form a flat or slightly curved surface, or umbel, which is distinctive of the umbellifer family and will help with identification. The fruit of hemlock is the most medicinally active part of the plant but is used only in minute homeopathic doses to relieve pain. In all other cases hemlock is deadly poisonous, especially its green, almost ripe seeds, and should never be harvested or used for any form of self-treatment.

Convallaria majalis LILY OF THE VALLEY

A hardy perennial, lily of the valley will grow in any soil but it thrives in humus-rich, moist earth such as that found in woodlands. This popular garden plant has white flowers that are drooping and bell shaped and emit a lovely, sweet smell. In autumn the lily produces bright red spherical berries that are highly toxic and can cause paralysis and respiratory failure.

Children, in particular, should be warned against touching or eating these attractive fruits.

Although all parts of the lily are extremely poisonous and should never be used for self-medication, some parts are used by herbalists for their beneficial action on the heart. The lily encourages a slow, regular heartbeat, in an action similar to that of foxglove.

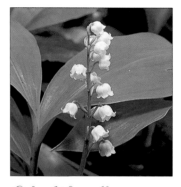

Lily of the valley

Digitalis purpurea FOXGLOVE

This hardy biennial, also considered a short-lived perennial, produces pink, mauve, red, or white trumpet-shaped flowers with spotted interiors. Found on wasteland and in gardens, all parts of the foxglove are highly toxic when taken internally, yet from this plant comes one of the most widely used and universally recognized heart drugs, digitoxin. Paradoxically, one of the symptoms of

digitalis poisoning is an irregular heart action. Other symptoms may include abdominal pain, stomach irritation, nausea, tremors, and even death.

Although the deep green oval leaves are sometimes prescribed as treatment for epilepsy and tumors, because of the danger of poisoning it is illegal to give foxglove as an internal preparation unless you are a qualified doctor.

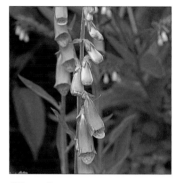

Foxglove

Hyoscyamus niger HENBANE

A woody-stemmed herb found mainly on wasteland and in sandy areas, henbane is extremely poisonous and foul smelling. All parts of the herb are covered in a fine down, and the flowers are pale yellow and pitcher shaped, with purple veins.

Henbane has a violent action that can result in palpitations, respiratory failure, delirium, hallucinations, and death. Used by professional herbalists, however, this herb can be useful in the treatment of

digestive, urinary tract, and asthmatic spasms. The sticky gray-green leaves also have pain-relieving properties that can reduce muscular spasms and induce a deep, healing sleep.

Henbane is widely used in herbalism, homeopathy, and conventional medicine, with the dosage carefully monitored. The essential oil is sometimes used in creams and liniments for relieving rheumatism and treating scar tissue.

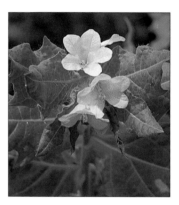

Henbane

Ilex aquifolium HOLLY

Found mostly in parks, gardens, and woodlands, holly is a popular Christmas plant because of its bright red winter berries and shiny rich green leaves. The berries of the holly are toxic, however, and can cause serious bouts of vomiting and diarrhea. This can be particularly dangerous for children, who may find the berries appealing. In professional use, the leaves are infused to help treat

colds and coughs, and they have diuretic properties that relieve urinary infections. They are also used as a fever remedy and have some therapeutic action in the treatment of jaundice and rheumatism.

Despite its many applications, holly should be used medicinally only under strict professional supervision and should never be used as a self-help treatment or for children.

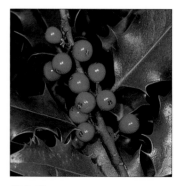

Holly

Cytisus Laburnum LABURNUM

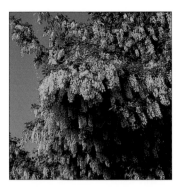

Laburnum

A small deciduous tree, laburnum can be found on mountainsides and in gardens and parks. It produces small yellow flowers in long, drooping groups, which inspire one of its common names, golden chain, and in autumn, brown seed pods that cluster along the stems.

All parts of the tree are poisonous, but particularly the unripe berries and the seed pods, so it is important that children be warned not to eat them. Symptoms of poisoning with laburnum include stomach cramps, severe vomiting, sweating, dilated pupils, respiratory failure, dizziness, and convulsions.

In homeopathic medicine a preparation of the leaves and flowers is used to relieve neurological and digestive disorders. Laburnum should never be used for self-treatment.

Lobelia inflata LOBELIA

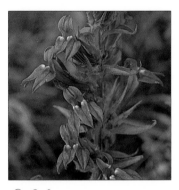

Lobelia

Also known as Indian tobacco, this plant contains certain extracts that are added to antismoking mixtures, and they have a taste similar to that of tobacco.

A popular house and garden plant in North America and western Europe, *Lobelia inflata* produces small, pretty, spiky lavender-blue flowers between June and October and has finely serrated, long, narrow leaves.

More toxic than other members of the lobelia family (Lobeliaceae), Indian tobacco has an emetic and expectorant action and is used in homeopathic remedies to treat asthma.

The symptoms of lobelia poisoning include nausea and vomiting, diarrhea, difficulty in breathing, headache, sweating and shivering, dizziness, irregular heartbeat, and convulsions.

Solanum dulcamara BITTERSWEET

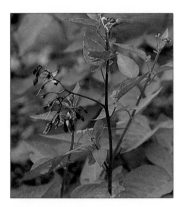

Bittersweet

A shrubby and aggressive climber, bittersweet has several other common names, including nightshade, bittersweet nightshade, felonwort, and violet bloom. It is an attractive plant with heart-shaped leaves and pretty star-shaped flowers, purple with yellow anthers.

The name bittersweet comes from its bright red berries, which at first taste bitter, then unpleasantly sweet. Most commonly found in woodlands and on streambanks, the plant is highly toxic and can cause diarrhea, nausea, vomiting, and dilated pupils.

Bittersweet is prescribed by herbalists and homeopaths as a liver tonic and an asthma treatment and can be applied topically to relieve skin disorders, such as acne, chronic exzema, and warts. The toxic bittersweet stems also have both diuretic and antirheumatic properties but should never be used as a home remedy.

Taxus baccata YEW

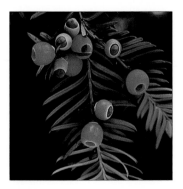

Yew

A slow-growing evergreen shrub or small tree, the yew has flattened dark green leaves but does not bear cones like other needled evergreens. In autumn it bears fruit that consists of a seed partially enclosed in a fleshy bright red cup when ripe. Strangely, the red cup is the only part of the yew that is not poisonous (it is sweet and edible), but the seeds and leaves are very toxic. Mild yew poisoning can cause gastroenteritis, vertigo, and vomiting, while larger doses can result in asphyxiation and cardiac arrest.

A tincture of fresh yew leaves is used in homeopathy to treat arthritis, gout, rheumatism, urinary tract infections, and heart and liver conditions. At one time yew was used by herbalists to treat a variety of conditions, but today it is widely considered too toxic.

MISAPPLICATION AND OVERDOSING

*The most common problems in herbal treatment are
not side effects—these are rare with herbs that are correctly
administered in therapeutic doses—but misapplication.*

Self-diagnosis is always potentially dangerous, and with herbal medicine even more so because the therapy can be subtle. Two apparently similar complaints may require different remedies, and the wrong herb may exacerbate a problem.

Some people will have an allergic reaction to certain herbs, often to a group of them that are related botanically, and may get a rash or a headache. If you have a history of allergies, start carefully when taking herbal remedies. Take a low dose of one herb by itself for a few days, rather than a mixture. If you are planning to apply an herb exter-

nally, do a patch test first. Try the remedy for a day or two on an area of skin that is not inflamed or irritated, to see if that herb gives you any adverse reactions.

If you do get a reaction, stop taking the herb. If the reaction is immediate and external, such as a rash, wash the area thoroughly with clean, warm water and pat dry. If other reactions occur, such as vomiting or chest pains, seek immediate medical advice.

Never try to relieve extreme allergic reactions with other untested herbs; you may exacerbate the symptoms. If you suffer a reaction, seek professional advice.

MAINTAINING SAFE LEVELS

The following remedies are safe as long as the dosage, duration of use, and rest periods are adhered to. The rest periods will ensure that there is not a dangerous buildup of the active constituents in your system. It is recommended that you obtain professional advice before embarking on a course of treatment.

NAME	MAXIMUM DAILY DOSE	DURATION (WEEKS)	REST PERIOD (WEEKS)	CONTRAINDICATIONS/CAUTIONS
Bearberry (*Arctostaphylos uva-ursi*)	3 g	2	2	May cause kidney disease if taken for a long time.
Blood root (*Sanguinaria canadensis*)	0.5 g	2	1	Follow professional advice. Avoid during pregnancy/lactation.
Broom (*Cytisus scoparius*)	3 g	2	1	Follow professional advice.
Cascara sagrada (*Cascara sagrada*)	3 g	1	2	Use for a few days at a time before bed.
Comfrey (*Symphytum officinalis*)	3 g	4	4	Use leaves only for internal use.
Ginseng (*Panax ginseng*)	2 g	12	4	May cause menstrual problems, nervous tension, heart disease. Avoid with caffeine.
Licorice (*Glycyrrhiza glabra*)	4 g	2	1	May cause hypertension.
Lignum vitae (*Guaiacum officinalis*)	2 g	4	2	May cause acute inflammation or allergy.
Pokeroot (*Phytolacca americana*)	0.3 g	2	2	Follow professional advice. Avoid during pregnancy.
Senna (*Cassia* species)	2 g	1	3	Not for colicky constipation. Avoid during pregnancy.
Tansy (*Tanacetum vulgare*)	1 g	2	2	Follow professional advice. Avoid during pregnancy.

OVERDOSING

Overdoses of toxic herbs are obviously dangerous, but even some milder herbs can have a cumulative ill effect and are best taken for short periods only. Others that are quite safe over long periods in therapeutic dosages can still cause unpleasant sensations or medical complications if taken in too large a dose. Always check to see if your chosen herbal remedy has a maximum safe dosage or is known to have any contraindications. Also, bear in mind that some herbs may be perfectly safe for most people but are contraindicated for specific conditions, such as pregnancy or hypertension. If in doubt, always seek professional advice.

The best way to choose the right herb is to find one that is commonly recommended for your condition and then to find out as much as you can about it. Pay attention to your whole range of symptoms and the range of actions attributed to the herb, and always take the recommended dose for the period of time that is advised.

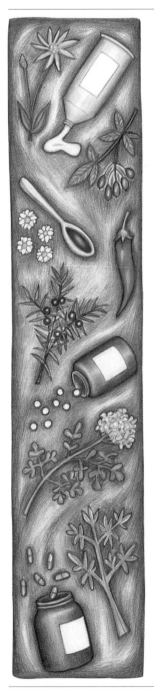

DAILY DOSES

The chart below lists a number of commonly available herbs that require particular care. Although all are generally available and safe when properly used, you must pay close attention to the dosage. Never exceed the daily dose. Stop treatment and consult your herbalist if you suffer any negative effects.

NAME	MAXIMUM DAILY DOSE	CONTRAINDICATIONS/CAUTIONS
Barberry (*Berberis vulgaris*)	2 g	Avoid during pregnancy.
Black cohosh (*Cimicifuga racemosa*)	1 g	Follow professional advice. Avoid during pregnancy.
Blue cohosh (*Caulophyllum thalictroides*)	1 g	Avoid during pregnancy, until labor.
Blue flag (*Iris versicolor*)	2 g	Discontinue in cases of digestive irritation.
Cayenne (*Capsicum annuum*)	120 mg	Avoid with gastric hyperacidity (acid indigestion).
Celery seed (*Apium graveolens*)	3 g	Avoid during pregnancy.
Feverfew (*Tanacetum parthenium*)	1 g	Avoid during pregnancy.
Figwort (*Scrophularia nodosa*)	5 g	Avoid with tachycardia (rapid heartbeat).
Goldenseal (*Hydrastis canadensis*)	2 g	Avoid during pregnancy. Do not give to children.
Hops (*Humulus lupulus*)	1 g	Avoid during depressive illness.
Juniper (*Juniperus communis*)	2 g	Avoid during pregnancy or with kidney disease.
Maté (*Ilex paraguariensis*)	4 g	Stimulating; treat like strong coffee.
Mugwort (*Artemisia vulgaris*)	2 g	Avoid during pregnancy.
Oats (*Avena sativa*)	4 g	Avoid if gluten sensitive.
Pasque flower (*Pulsatilla pratensis*)	0.3 g	Do not use when fresh.
Pennyroyal (*Mentha pulegium*)	3 g	Avoid during pregnancy.
Queen's delight (*Stillingia sylvatica*)	2 g	Do not use after two years of storage.
Rue (*Ruta graveolens*)	1 g	Avoid during pregnancy.
Sage (*Salvia officinalis*)	3 g	Avoid during pregnancy.
Sassafras (*Sassafras albidum*)	3 g	Do not use the essential oil internally.
Sweet flag (*Acorus calamus*)	2 g	Keep within stated dose; avoid isolated oil.
Thuja (*Thuja occidentalis*)	3 g	Avoid during pregnancy.
Wild lettuce (*Lactuca virosa*)	3 g	High doses can be dangerous.
Wormwood (*Artemisia absinthium*)	2 g	Avoid during pregnancy.

TREATMENT AND SELF-DIAGNOSIS

Herbal treatments often complement conventional medical care but can also interfere with it. Always inform your doctor or therapist of any medicines you are taking.

Many common health problems—colds, headaches, insomnia, and indigestion—are minor, and few people consider professional treatment to be necessary for them. Other disorders, such as hay fever, may be more of a nuisance than a serious health concern, yet for all these conditions there is effective herbal treatment. For symptoms that need urgent attention (see page 66), you should see your general practitioner or go to the nearest hospital emergency room or department. Medical professionals can refer you for tests, if necessary, or send you to a specialist who can deal with the problem.

Some less urgent conditions can be treated by a properly trained herbalist. These would include doctors of oriental medicine and of naturopathy. If your problem needs further treatment, an herbal specialist will ask you to consult your primary care physician and may contact the doctor or write a letter for you to take along.

IS IT SAFE TO TAKE HERBS WITH MEDICINAL DRUGS?

If a condition is serious enough to require medical treatment, you should not add to or modify the treatment without professional supervision. In general, an herbalist or pharmacognosist will know more about interactions between herbs and drugs than an orthodox doctor, because few physicians are familiar with medicinal herbs. But, in fact, relatively little is known about interactions between drugs and herbs because these effects are not studied in standard tests, and there is no reporting system for recording such interactions should they occur (unlike interactions of two or more drugs, which doctors report to pharmaceutical companies so that the information can be relayed to other medical professionals.)

If you are seeing an herbalist as well as taking medications prescribed by your doctor, you should bring any prescription medicines with you to the herbal consultation, and the herbalist should take them into account. You should also inform your physician if you are seeing an herbalist. It is not just courteous but also sensible to keep everyone involved in your treatment aware of the others. Good practitioners of alternative medicine will encourage you to inform your doctor or will do so themselves.

CHOOSING A PRACTITIONER

A good health care practitioner, whether a medical doctor, herbalist, or other therapist, is always eager to learn more about health care and will be genuinely concerned about you and your condition. He or she should be willing to discuss all aspects of your treatment with you, giving you a clear description of the causes of your condition and what is likely to happen and why. If you get a strong impression that your practitioner has hardly listened to a word you have said or has dismissed your worries, you should think about looking for someone else.

Reactions to both herbs and drugs always carry a certain amount of unpredictability. You may get side effects with one medicine or another, and new aspects of your condi-

Mint and Lemongrass Tea
to soothe indigestion

2 tbsp dried peppermint
1 tbsp dried, chopped lemongrass
1 tbsp crushed fennel seeds
1 tbsp dried chamomile flowers

■ Place all the herbs in an airtight can and shake to mix them thoroughly.
■ To make the tea, put 1 tsp of the mix in a cup and add hot but not boiling water. Leave to steep for 5 minutes.
■ Take 1 cup after rich, heavy meals to soothe indigestion.

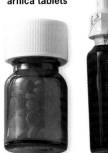

Witch hazel lotion

Bach rescue remedy

Homeopathic arnica tablets

Arnica ointment

HOLISTIC FIRST AID
A simple first-aid kit that includes herbal and homeopathic remedies can provide immediate relief for an injury before medical help is available. For shock, Bach flower rescue remedy or homeopathic arnica tablets can help. For minor burns and sunburn, distilled witch hazel or aloe vera will relieve pain. Bruises and sprains can be eased with arnica ointment, but it should be applied only to unbroken skin.

tion may come to light. Your treatment may therefore change significantly over time. If you develop serious side effects with a particular medicine or suffer a series of different reactions or unexplained changes in symptoms, you should contact your herbal specialist or physician. If your concerns are pushed aside, consider a change of practitioner. A health care practitioner who suits one patient may, for reasons of personality or professional strengths and weaknesses, not suit another. You must be able to trust whoever is treating you, both as a person and as a therapist, not only because he or she is responsible for your health but also because, without that trust,

HERBAL REMEDIES VERSUS OVER-THE-COUNTER AIDS

Many over-the-counter medicines, especially syrups and lozenges sold to remedy coughs and sore throats, are highly sugared and have limited real medicinal value.

This is not to say that many such medicines will not relieve immediate symptoms of minor illnesses, but that many homemade herbal remedies can be used to treat the same conditions and will have a more beneficial overall medicinal effect.

For conditions in which medical help is needed, herbal first aid will give just as effective immediate relief as most conventional over-the-counter first-aid treatments.

you will be less receptive and your treatment may then be less effective. If you don't trust your therapist, you may stop the treatment too early to derive any benefit.

SELF-DIAGNOSIS
Going to your doctor with a common complaint such as diarrhea or a cold is usually unnecessary because these symptoms tend to disappear after a few days, even if left untreated. In such instances, self-diagnosis is often perfectly adequate, and the use of herbs to alleviate any pain and hasten the healing process is fine. However, if mild symptoms last for more than a few days or become increasingly worse, they may signal a more serious underlying illness, and you should consult a professional.

Skin problems
There are many herbs that can help alleviate the effects of certain skin disorders; examples are red clover or figwort for psoriasis and yellow dock or burdock for eczema. Self-diagnosis, however, may not be sufficient. Contact dermatitis, for instance, may not be relieved by herbal treatment if the cause is an allergic reaction to some metal, such as nickel in your watch or jewelry. Likewise, contact with an allergen like feathers or grass may be causing the skin condition.

Irritant eczema could be caused by a shower gel, dishwashing liquid, or other detergent and will clear up without the use of herbal remedies. Not only would herbs be redundant in all the above cases, but the treatment might mask the underlying need to rid yourself of the irritant or allergen.

Vomiting
Any sustained or prolonged vomiting should be treated professionally. Although herbs such as chamomile and fennel can relieve nausea and vomiting, it is important that you rule out possible causes such as a perforated duodenal ulcer or gastroenteritis before you begin herbal treatment. Many digestive complaints are symptoms of other, more serious problems.

Chest pains
Mint or fennel may help relieve the pain of indigestion but sudden chest pains may, in fact, be caused by muscular problems or be a precursor to a heart attack, in which case you should seek immediate medical advice.

An Indigestion Sufferer

Self-treatment for persistent digestive problems without professional advice can be hazardous because such pains may be symptoms of a serious disorder such as colitis or appendicitis. If you have abdominal pain or indigestion that persists, it is vital that you seek medical attention to determine the underlying cause.

Tim is a 23-year-old legal secretary with a busy social life. He is careful about his weight but tends to eat a lot of snacks and fast food. He has always had good health, apart from occasional constipation.

After two bouts of abdominal discomfort within a few weeks of each other, Tim thought he might have irritable bowel syndrome and decided to relax more and to cut down on fast foods. He also tried peppermint tea, which seemed to help. Then Tim had another bout one evening, which was so bad he couldn't eat and had to lie down.

The most recent episode was much worse, with extreme pain emanating from his lower right side and a slight fever. This time he was nauseated and realized he had to take action.

WHAT SHOULD TIM DO?

With such serious symptoms, Tim needs to call a doctor right away. His attempt to improve his lifestyle and diet was a good approach for general improvement in well-being and, as a step for dealing with abdominal discomfort, was perfectly sensible. Taking peppermint tea was also fine for symptomatic relief but not as a substitute for correct diagnosis and treatment.

If Tim cannot obtain an immediate appointment with his doctor, he should seek help at the nearest hospital. The symptoms he is experiencing now are typical of acute appendicitis, and if he ignores the condition, his appendix could rupture and lead to peritonitis, a life-threatening inflammation.

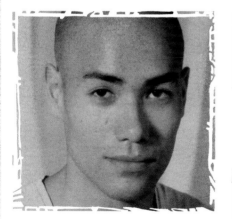

LIFESTYLE
Busy people often ignore signs of illness, but prolonged problems should be treated professionally.

HEALTH
Some serious medical problems can be masked by general symptoms and easily misdiagnosed.

SELF-HELP
Be aware that self-diagnosis and home treatment should not be continued if there is no sign of improvement within a day or so. This is most important when symptoms worsen.

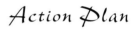

Action Plan

HEALTH
Consult a doctor before symptoms become debilitating. Fast action can often prevent serious consequences and bring a swift recovery.

SELF-HELP
Strive for a healthy, balanced diet, including limiting intake of fast foods, to help reduce the risk of major disorders.

LIFESTYLE
Attend to illness properly. Quick-fix remedies may lead to more serious complications.

HOW THINGS TURNED OUT FOR TIM

Tim called a friend because he realized that something was very wrong. His friend took him to a nearby emergency room, where he was diagnosed with acute appendicitis. Tim's appendix was removed the next morning, and two weeks later he was back at work.

Tim is still eating healthier foods and regularly goes to a yoga class for relaxation. The experience has made him much readier to seek professional help when symptoms persist.

EMERGENCIES

If any of the following signs develop, seek medical attention right away and do not try herbal or other self-help remedies.

▶ *Severe pain or pressure in the center chest that lasts more than 2 minutes*

▶ *Sudden severe headache*

▶ *Body temperature rises to 39.4°C (103°F)*

▶ *Fever of any degree accompanied by severe headache, stiff neck, swelling of the throat, or mental confusion*

▶ *Unexplained dizziness or loss of consciousness*

▶ *Sudden weakness or numbness on one side of the body*

▶ *Rapid weak pulse and rapid, shallow, and irregular breathing*

Headaches

While feverfew, rosemary, and chamomile are good for soothing a headache, the real problem may be as simple as bad posture, resulting in muscle strain in your neck. Correcting your sitting position during the day could be all that is necessary to relieve your headaches. Likewise, poor lighting when reading or unsuitable prescription glasses may be the cause of headaches, and addressing those problems rather than treating the symptoms makes the taking of herbs unnecessary. An especially severe headache that comes on suddenly or one that is accompanied by a high fever, stiff neck, confusion, blurred vision, or partial paralysis usually indicates a serious condition and requires immediate medical care.

WHEN NOT TO USE HERBS

Some symptoms of serious illness demand immediate action. An understanding of the strengths and weaknesses of herbal remedies will help you to choose the most appropriate available treatment.

If your house catches fire, you may experience severe nervous tension. You are, however, unlikely to take a remedy like valerian tea but would instead try to put out the fire or escape! In the same way, you must know how to react to your medical symptoms effectively in order to minimize any danger to your health. Although herbs are usually more gentle in their action than many of the analgesics and decongestants you can buy at a pharmacy, they can still mask, or at least ameliorate, symptoms of serious illness. This is particularly true for digestive problems and some respiratory conditions. It is therefore important to be aware of symptoms that may indicate serious trouble before using any form of self-medication.

PROTRACTED SYMPTOMS

There are certain symptoms that do not need to be brought immediately to the attention of a doctor, but if they persist for more than a few days, you should seek help. These include sudden weight loss without apparent cause; a constant thirst for no reason; having a mole increase in size or thickness, change color, or become itchy or bleed easily; a change in your voice—becoming husky or hoarse; a change or lump in your breasts, nipples, or scrotum; constant indigestion or acid belching; and feeling tired without good reason. Also, the passing of blood, whether in stools, urine, vomit, or sputum, requires prompt attention.

OTHER SERIOUS SYMPTOMS

Apart from the above symptoms for which medical treatment is imperative, there are some general rules to follow. If the problem is a familiar one that normally resolves itself—a chesty cough following a cold or a headache when tired, for example—use self-treatment and wait for it to pass.

Signs that you should seek professional help include the failure of a mild condition to respond to herbal treatment within a reasonable period of time—generally two weeks but, in the case of feverish illnesses and other conditions such as continuous headaches or headaches made worse by coughing, a week; a worsening of the condition; or the development of new symptoms.

Any sudden breathing problem; loss of vision, hearing, or feeling; or the development of an exceptionally high temperature should be treated as very serious and medical attention sought immediately.

CAUTION

Children are often unaware of the severity of their symptoms. You must judge when a doctor is needed. If in doubt, call the doctor anyway. The signs below are considered serious.

▶ *Sudden drowsiness or breathing problems, such as gulping, gasping for air, wheezing, or the inability to drink or speak*

▶ *Pain on breathing, violet spots that do not fade when pressed, weakness, confusion*

▶ *Abdominal swelling and tenderness accompanied by fever*

▶ *Severe diarrhea and vomiting at the same time*

▶ *The inability to sit up or bend the head forward*

▶ *Bleeding from any body opening, like ears, nose, or mouth*

▶ *Blood in the stool or urine*

▶ *Body temperature rises to 38°C (100.5°F) in a baby under 3 months, 39.4°C (103°F) in a child of any other age*

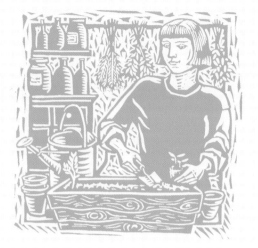

HERBAL PREPARATIONS

Many professional herbalists still make their own remedies, a tradition that has survived for centuries. Commercially produced herbal preparations require large-scale horticultural and complex manufacturing processes with strict quality controls, but quite a few herbs can also be safely and successfully cultivated in pots and gardens to be used as home remedies.

GROWING YOUR OWN HERBS

Anyone with a garden or a sunny windowsill can grow herbs. Most are very self-sufficient plants and, given just a little care and attention, will thrive almost anywhere.

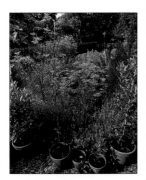

HERBS AT HOME
An herb garden can be established in pots or beds in almost any garden spot and doesn't require a lot of space. The closer your herbs are to the kitchen, the better, as this will allow you to tend and harvest them with ease.

The advantages of growing your own herbs are numerous. You do not need much space to create an herb garden; even a selection of herbs grown in a window box will provide a small annual harvest. Many herbs are very attractive and have culinary uses, so even if you do not wish to make medicines from them, they will make a useful addition to your home.

ESTABLISHING YOUR OWN HERB GARDEN

Having your own herb garden gives you the opportunity to use the herbs immediately after they have been harvested, which can be important when making medical preparations at home. Growing culinary herbs in a flowerbed or in pots on a patio or win-

dowsill near the kitchen also makes them accessible and easy to tend, but choose a place away from busy streets in order to avoid contamination by exhaust fumes.

Correct identification is absolutely essential when collecting plants for herbal remedies. Cutting the wrong herb for home use can at best make your medicine ineffective, but at worst it could lead to poisoning. If you grow your own herbs, buy seeds and seedlings from reputable suppliers so you will always know what you are planting and using. In addition, medicinal plants are becoming increasingly rare in the wild, and most countries place restrictions on which plants may be picked. Growing your own supply of herbs instead of gathering them will help to preserve herbs growing in the

PLANNING AN HERB GARDEN

Before you plant your herb garden, consider the space you have for your herbs and bear in mind which plants you want to grow.

Plot out your space and mark the areas that are best suited to your chosen plants. Identify the sunniest, shadiest, and moistest areas of your garden and plant your herbs accordingly. If you are going to gather your herbs frequently, make sure that you can reach them easily without trampling other plants.

PLANNING YOUR GARDEN
Try to envisage how your garden will look once the plants have matured, and how your herbs will work around fixed features such as trees and ponds.

Shady areas
Beds found around the base of trees and shadowed by walls or buildings are ideal for woodland herbs that can thrive in shade. These include mint and lady's mantle.

Damp areas
Position water-loving plants such as bergamot and peppermint in any parts of your garden that naturally retain water, such as hollows or soil beside ponds.

Partial sun areas
Elecampane, marigold, and borage are herbs that enjoy partial sunlight. Areas that are shaded for parts of the day or that allow dappled light through are ideal.

Sunny areas
Many herbs adore bright sunshine, and the sunniest area of your garden should contain your main herb bed. Plant herbs like hyssop and lavender here.

wild. If you take cuttings from plants, be careful that you damage the plant as little as possible. When buying seeds, make sure they are dry and free from mold.

GETTING STARTED
Before you start planting, plan your herb garden carefully, taking into consideration space restrictions, the condition of the soil, and what direction your garden faces.

Most herbs prefer a sunny, sheltered spot with well-drained soil, but you should choose herbs that suit your garden site. For warm, south-facing areas choose sun-loving plants like thyme, rosemary, and chamomile. You can grow herbs like peppermint and marsh mallow if your soil retains water.

Put tall plants like elecampane and mullein at the back of your border and let creepers such as thyme and lady's mantle spread along the edge. If grown in the right conditions, herbs make few demands and need only a little basic care.

ANNUALS
Annual plants have to be grown from seed each spring. Herbs that belong to this group flower and produce seeds and then die within their one-year life cycle. Most can be sown straight into the soil in mid- to late spring. Some herbs, like parsley, germinate slowly and may need to be kept indoors until the seedlings are strong enough to be

GROWING HERBS IN POTS
Herbs can thrive in containers, but do not like too much direct sunlight because the heat dries them out too quickly and saps their vitality. They need to be watered more often than their garden companions to keep them in good condition.

The key to success for healthy herbs in pots and window boxes lies in a good position, adequate drainage, and a good-quality potting mixture. Choose a sunny but partially sheltered spot and make sure you plant the herbs in containers that will accommodate them comfortably. If your containers are lightweight, they can be easily moved indoors to give tender plants protection during the winter months.

Growing Herbs from Seeds and Cuttings

To ensure successful seed or root cultivation, make sure that seeds and roots are healthy and that any damage is kept to a minimum. Soil should be high quality, preferably loam-based, and should be kept moist. Any cuts to roots should be clean and neat, while seeds should be planted with adequate room for growth.

transferred to the garden. Many annuals do not grow very tall and can easily be planted among the perennials in your garden. Most of them are prolific seed producers and often tend to self-seed—that is, they disperse their seeds themselves. Many of them also make very good plants for window boxes and containers because they have attractive flowers. Easy-to-grow annuals include marigold and basil.

BIENNIALS
Biennials have a life cycle of two years, producing foliage in the first year and flowers and seeds in the second. Herbs in this category should be harvested in their second year, just before they die. They need to be sown again the following year. Biennial plants can grow quite tall, which you need to bear in mind when planning your herb garden. Among the herbs that belong to this group are angelica and cumin.

PERENNIALS
Perennial herbs will establish themselves and thrive for several years if grown in the right location. Some, like thyme and sage, are evergreen plants and keep their leaves during the winter months. Others, like feverfew and lady's mantle, die back in autumn and produce new growth each spring. Grow perennials in the largest bed in your garden and give them enough space to expand and reach their full size. Perennials have their own growing cycle but, unlike annuals and biennials, do not need to be replaced frequently. They will thrive for three to four years before they need to be divided and replanted in a new location to give them enough room to keep them healthy. Cut back evergreen perennials each autumn to encourage vigorous growth the following year. Attractive perennials include wood betony, elecampane, and

Sow seeds in small pots and keep under a piece of glass or clear plastic until growth begins to show.

Root cuttings can be taken from woody herbs such as rosemary. Take a strong shoot, away from the main stem, and dip it into hormone rooting powder before planting.

Rosemary cutting

Rooting powder

A loam-based planting mix is most suitable for potting herbs. If using a peat-based formula, add one part sand to five parts soil to improve drainage.

A dibble will help to make holes of the correct depth and width.

Label plants clearly to avoid confusion later on.

Feverfew
camomile

The Horticulturist

Horticulture is the science of cultivating plants for both food and display. It includes the commercial growing of such crops as fruits, flowers, and vegetables, as well as all aspects of landscape gardening.

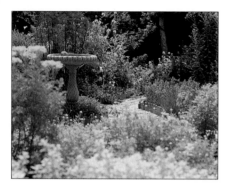

THE BEAUTY OF HERBS
Many herbs are cultivated for their beauty as well as their medicinal and culinary uses. Herbs have been an attractive feature in ornamental gardens for centuries.

THE HORTICULTURIST
Understanding the often surprising relationships between different plants is a fundamental aspect of the horticulturist's trade. Planting marigolds next to pole beans, for example, is a natural, organic way to control black fly.

Modern horticulturists treat their vocation as a science and employ methods of propagating and harvesting plants that are way beyond what was known only a hundred years ago. However, traditional methods of growing crops are still used in organic horticulture, which is particularly important for the cultivation of medicinal plants.

What does horticulture involve?
Horticulture is divided into two areas: commercial and environmental. Commercial horticulture includes the large-scale growing and harvesting of fruit and vegetable crops for consumption as well as the cultivation of flowers for decorative purposes. This involves propagating the crop from seeds, thinning out seedlings, and looking after the plants while they grow. Horticultural workers use fertilizers, pesticides, and herbicides to obtain the maximum yield from their crops. The timing of a harvest is also very important in commercial horticulture because produce must be in peak condition when sold.

Environmental horticulture includes the planning, planting, and maintenance of public and private gardens, parks, and other open spaces. Propagation and plant care are similar to those of commercial horticulture, but harvesting is not an important part of the work because the plants are not grown for consumption.

Do horticulturists grow herbs?
Many culinary herbs that are available in supermarkets and garden centers have been grown by professional horticulturists using intensive cultivation methods—that is, they are given fertilizers to make them grow faster in order to meet popular demand. In addition, they are treated routinely with herbicides and pesticides to keep them disease free. Herbs from such crops are acceptable for culinary use but are not usually suitable for use as herbal medicines. Organically grown herbs are preferred for medicinal use because they carry no pesticide residues.

How are medicinal plants cultivated?

The best herbal preparations are made from plants that have been grown organically. Organic gardening is a relatively new branch of horticulture, but the methods organic gardeners use to grow their crops are based on traditional and long-established practices.

In organic horticulture, plants are grown without the help of synthetic fertilizers or pesticides, most of which are poisonous. Instead, organic gardeners take advantage of nature's ability to establish a healthy environment in which plants can thrive without the need for much intervention. This involves methods such as crop rotation, companion planting, and biological pest control. Insects like ladybirds and hoverflies, for example, feed on certain common pests and so are welcomed as natural pest control agents.

Crops are rotated frequently to keep the soil in good condition, which is important for healthy root growth. Organic horticulturists also know that certain plants grow well together and others do not, and they plant their crops accordingly. Thus, for example, an organic farmer knows that the smell of onions deters the carrot fly and will therefore plant onions among carrots rather than use chemicals to preserve the crop.

Using these methods for herbs ensures that the plants can develop their active constituents fully and are free from chemicals that might interfere with their healing powers.

Do organic horticulturists need special training?

Horticulture requires academic knowledge as well as a range of practical skills. Horticultural colleges teach sciences like biology and botany, to give students a theoretical background, and also provide training in hands-on subjects such as crop management, which involves propagation and harvesting. Many colleges also offer courses in organic horticulture to teach the special methods needed for this branch.

Origins

The cultivation of plants for food and medicine can be traced back thousands of years. Ancient civilizations like the Aztecs of Mexico and the Egyptians in Africa grew grains for food, herbs for medicine, and flowers for use in celebrations and rituals. Even then, cultivation of plants was carefully planned and skillfully executed to obtain the best possible harvest.

The Middle Ages in Great Britain saw a vast interest in the cultivation of herbs, coupled with an aesthetic pleasure in beautiful gardens. Elizabethan gardens of the 16th century continue to influence the design of public and private gardens today.

Settlers in North America brought with them plants from their native countries and learned from Indians how to cultivate and use local ones.

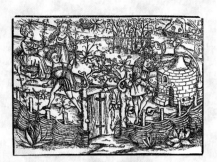

MEDIEVAL HERB GARDEN
The Middle Ages were an important time for horticulture in Europe. This period is famous for the kitchen and herb gardens of monasteries and royal palaces, where plants were grown for culinary and medicinal purposes.

Scientific discoveries of the 20th century shaped modern horticulture, which uses methods and techniques that allow plants to be cultivated on a much larger scale than ever before.

WHAT YOU CAN DO AT HOME

There are various methods of plant propagation that are easy to employ. Other than sowing seeds, two of the most popular techniques are to propagate from cuttings and by root division.

For the best cuttings, choose a healthy young plant and cut just below a leaf and stem joint with a clean, sharp knife. Try not to make more than one clean cut. Dip the cut stem in a good-quality rooting preparation, widely available in nurseries and hardware stores. Insert the stem into the ground near the plant and water well.

For propagation using root division, carefully divide a mature plant into smaller separate sections, making sure that each section has a reasonable amount of root attached. Then simply replant the sections as individual plants.

ROOT DIVISION
It is important to use a clean, sharp knife when dividing roots and take care that damage to the root is minimal.

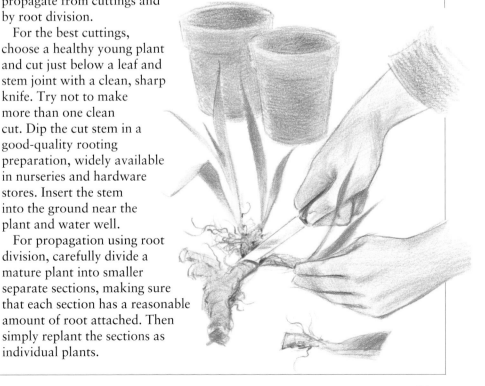

Herb Garden

You can create a small herb garden on your balcony or windowsill by planting a few flowering pots or a window box with easy-to-grow plants such as basil, thyme, and nasturtium.

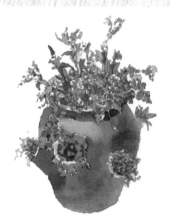

TERRA-COTTA STRAWBERRY POT
Terra-cotta pots are beautiful but dry out quickly. Soak them in water several hours before planting to prevent their taking moisture from newly potted plants.

Planting herbs in containers can be sensible for any kind of space—from a windowsill to a backyard—because it allows you to move herbs to follow the sun or keep them out of the wind. It's best not to overcrowd containers; herbs need ample room for their roots. Keep perennial herbs in their nursery pots within a window box. This will protect them through the winter and prevent their roots from taking over too much of the box.

PLANTING A WINDOW BOX

Window boxes made from plastic or fiberglass are durable and retain moisture well, but do not have the esthetic appeal of terra-cotta. Other options include wooden troughs and wooden or tin tubs.

To get started, you will need your chosen window box, a good-quality potting mixture, and a selection of herbs. You will also need clay pot shards or pebbles for lining the bottom of the container. These allow the root system free drainage and air circulation, so that you avoid waterlogging your container and rotting the roots of the herbs; they will have a better chance to mature.

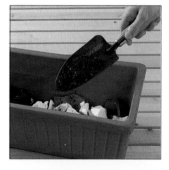

1 *Cover the container bottom with 2.5 cm (1 in) of pebbles or pot shards. Cover the pebbles with a layer of potting mixture. Keep perennials in their pots to protect them when you replace annuals after they die down; plant annuals directly in the soil.*

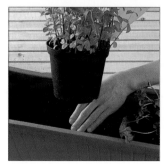

2 *Place perennials with their pots in the container and fill the remaining space with potting soil to within 2.5 cm (1 in) of the rim. Always position taller plants at the back of the box.*

3 *Plant the annuals, one at a time, directly in the soil between the perennials. Put in each herb so that its roots are well covered with earth, taking care to press firmly around the base of each herb with your fingertips in order to anchor it in the soil. Gently water the newly planted box to settle the herbs in and wash any soil from the leaves.*

CUTTING AND DRYING HERBS

All herbs have an optimum time when their leaves, flowers, seeds, or roots should be harvested. To ensure the best herbal preparations, harvest herbs only at the recommended times.

Depending on the particular plant and the intended use, an herbal preparation can be made from leaves, stems, bark, flowers, roots, or seeds. In culinary usage an herb usually consists of the leaves and sometimes the flowers of a plant, and a spice is derived from the seeds, bark, or root. Examples of culinary herbs are sage, parsley, basil, thyme, and rosemary, also dill and cilantro (the leaves of the dill and coriander plants). Examples of spices are ginger (root), cinnamon (bark), and fennel, dill, cumin, and coriander (seeds).

Most herbs wilt soon after cutting and should be dried as soon as possible. Once dried, they will keep best in clean brown paper bags or dark glass containers away from direct sunlight.

LEAVES

The optimum time to gather leaves is on a dry day after the morning dew has evaporated. Aromatic herbs like rosemary, sage, and peppermint give off their fragrance, and with it their essential oils, in the midday sun; they should be cut just before noon, when their volatile oil content is at its peak.

Leaves are best harvested from young shoots up to the time of flowering. Choose healthy plants that are free of dirt, disease, and insect damage, taking care not to crush or bruise them.

Before drying, wipe off any soil but do not wash the leaves, as they are more likely to become moldy if left damp. (Better yet, hose or spritz them the night before cutting.) Cut herbs should be kept out of direct sunlight because it will spoil their quality and diminish their therapeutic actions. The best place to dry leaves is in a warm, dry, dark environment with reasonable ventilation. A drying temperature of around 24°C (75°F) is ideal. Most leaves take about a week to dry completely, but very succulent or very thick leaves may take up to four weeks. Remove leaves from their stems and spread them on paper (not newspaper, as the printing ink may stain the leaves) or a screen (see right), or tie the stems in small bunches and hang them upside down. In fine weather leaves can be dried outdoors in a sheltered, well-aired place like a balcony or porch.

FLOWERS

Harvest flowers when their healing properties are at their best—just after they have opened. Pick them in dry weather, before the midday heat. Choose undamaged flowers and avoid bruising the petals. After picking, keep flowers out of direct sunlight and in a cool place because they wilt quickly.

Most flowers are fragile and need to be handled carefully throughout the drying process. After cutting, spread them thinly on paper or muslin. Do not wash them, as this would destroy all but the toughest flower heads. Flowers will retain their color

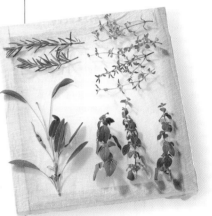

DRYING HERBS
Fine, rustproof mesh stretched over a wooden frame makes an ideal drying rack, allowing air to circulate thoroughly. Alternatively, bunches of stems can be hung over a length of string or wooden rod in a warm place. Pack stems loosely to let air circulate. Cover flower heads with a bag while drying to catch loose seeds and petals.

Separate dried stems over paper to catch seeds, leaves, and flowers.

Folding a crease into the paper first will make it easier to pour the loose herbs into storage jars.

if dried correctly but will fade if the temperature is too high. A room temperature of around 21°C (70°F) is generally ideal. Small flowers like chamomile take about a week to dry, while larger, thicker flowers such as marigolds can take up to three weeks to reach perfect dryness.

ROOTS

Roots should be collected in autumn, when the plant begins to store its therapeutic compounds belowground. Most roots that are used for medicinal purposes come from biennials or perennials and should be harvested in the plant's second or third year.

Dig up roots carefully without crushing them or making unnecessary cuts. Decide how much you will need to use and replant the rest where you found them. Never take the whole root of a perennial, as this denies the plant the chance to regrow.

Most roots, such as dandelion and burdock, can be scrubbed clean with water before drying, but others like valerian should be cleaned gently with a damp cloth because their active principles are contained in the outer layer, which must be retained.

Slice large, thick roots lengthwise into strips to aid drying. Roots dry better at higher temperatures than leaves or flowers because they are denser and tougher. Between 40° and 50°C (105° and 120°F) is ideal; a drying temperature should not exceed 60°C (140°F).

Roots can be dried in a dehydrating box (two to five days) or in the oven with the door open (two to three hours), but need to be turned occasionally. The temperature is important, but the flow of dry air is also a vital factor in drying. Check that your dehydrator has adequate airflow; the door should have holes or gaps in the bottom and top. When completely dry, roots will break easily in your hands.

SEEDS

Collect seeds when the seedpods of a plant are fully ripe. Ripe seed heads contain no green color and have a papery texture. Always harvest seeds on a warm, dry day and shake them into a paper bag or onto a tray. Ripe seeds should come off the heads easily. Make sure you save some of the seeds from annual plants for propagation, to ensure a good harvest the following year.

Seeds dry very quickly in airy, warm conditions, such as in a dehydrating box; they will be ready for storage after a week or two. The temperature for drying seeds is the same as for roots, but it is not advisable to dry seeds in the oven. Many seeds are collected for their aromatic properties, and drying at too high a temperature will evaporate the aromatic oils.

BARKS

The best time to collect the bark of trees is in damp weather, because it will peel off more easily when wet. Take the fresh bark from young trunks or branches, but never strip a whole ring of bark from around the tree's girth, because this may interfere with its feeding system and may also cause irreparable damage.

Check the stripped bark for insects and moss and remove them carefully with a damp cloth. Bark will dry more quickly in small pieces than in one large section.

Dry bark in a warm, dark, and airy place at the same temperature as for roots (about 50°C, or 120°F) until it feels dry and breaks easily. This may take from one to four weeks. Bark can also be dried in the oven, again at the same temperature as for roots: 40° to 50°C (105° to 120°F). Drying will take two to three hours.

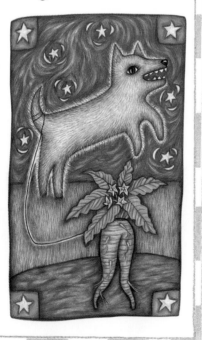

Herbal Myths

Mandrake, with its human-shaped root, is regarded in legend as an aphrodisiac and virility booster and has long been considered a supernatural being. The being was believed to emit a scream on uprooting, so chilling and powerful that it could kill the harvester.

To avoid such a death, harvesters would tie a dog to the root by its tail and let the dog suffer the screams. Uprooting was carried out at night to protect the power of the root, and this no doubt added to the superstitious myths surrounding the plant.

TYPES OF PREPARATION

Herbs can be used in many different ways. When choosing an herbal remedy, it helps to have some understanding of the various types of preparation that are possible.

Once you are aware of the different properties of herbs, you can decide on the best preparation for your needs. Some require significant time and special materials, while others simply need boiling water. Thorough sterilization of all utensils and storage containers is important. Sterilizing your equipment for 30 minutes before use will ensure that your preparations do not become contaminated and will lengthen the life of creams and syrups because they will less likely become moldy.

When choosing a remedy, it is important to know exactly what ailment you are going to treat (see Chapter 6) and the parts of the herb or herbs that you will need to obtain the desired effects (see Chapter 5).

INTERNAL PREPARATIONS

The majority of preparations for internal use are liquids that have the active ingredients of the herbs drawn into a solution. Whether water or alcohol based, liquid internal remedies are among the simplest herbal preparations and require little or no special equipment.

Infusions

Also called teas or tisanes, infusions are water-based extracts of plants that most often make use of the delicate parts, such as the flowers, leaves, and green stems. They are the best choice when a mild preparation is required, for example, a remedy for children or people who cannot tolerate alcohol. Infusions are also used for compresses when a mild external application is desired.

Infusions are made with water that has been boiled and then left to stand for 30 seconds. Typically, 25 g (1 oz) of dried herb or 50 g (1¾ oz) of fresh herb is used to make 600 ml (2½ cups) of tea. The procedure is to put the herb into a warmed china or glass—not metal—teapot, pour the hot water over it,

EQUIPMENT
Some preparations have clearly defined steps, just like recipes, so it is always best to have at hand all the equipment you will need before you begin. Some remedies like inhalations are quick to prepare but may become unusable if left to cool while you search for a towel to cover your head.

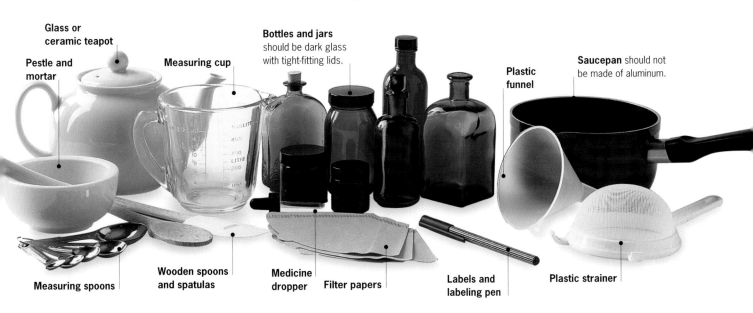

Glass or ceramic teapot

Pestle and mortar

Measuring cup

Bottles and jars should be dark glass with tight-fitting lids.

Plastic funnel

Saucepan should not be made of aluminum.

Measuring spoons

Wooden spoons and spatulas

Medicine dropper

Filter papers

Labels and labeling pen

Plastic strainer

Herbal Preparations

Both internal preparations (left) and external formulations (see far right) are tailored to treat specific ailments and as such must be prepared very carefully. It is a good idea to visualize your preparation to know how much to make and to take. An infusion, for example, is often the size of a cup of tea, while tinctures are taken by the teaspoonful.

then cover it and steep for 5 to 10 minutes, depending on the strength required. Strain and, if desired, sweeten with honey or brown sugar or flavor with fresh lemon juice. Sip it slowly while hot. The standard dosage for herbal teas is one cup two or three times a day for adults and half this amount for children under 12, unless stated otherwise.

An infusion is normally used immediately after preparation. It can be refrigerated for up to two days, but if there is any sign of spoiling, it must be discarded.

Some plants contain active constituents that are water soluble but are destroyed when heated. Herbs like marsh mallow and mullein contain large amounts of mucilage (see page 84) and need to be prepared as cold infusions. The quantities for cold infusions are the same as for hot ones. Soak the herb in cold water in a glass or china pot for 8 to 12 hours or overnight; strain and drink cold. Prepare a fresh infusion every day.

Decoctions

Like infusions, decoctions are water based but are made with the tougher plant parts, such as seeds, barks, and roots, which release their active constituents only if cut or broken into small pieces and simmered.

To prepare a decoction, use 25 g (1 oz) broken dried herb or 50 g (1¾ oz) chopped fresh herb to make 600 ml (2½ cups) of the decoction. Put the herb into an enamel or stainless-steel pan and cover with cold water and a tight-fitting lid. Slowly bring to a boil, then lower the heat and simmer for 15 minutes. Strain the liquid into another container. Sweeten with honey if desired and sip slowly while hot. The standard dose is half a cup three times a day for adults and half this amount for children under 12, unless stated otherwise.

Decoctions will keep for three days if refrigerated, but are at their most effective when freshly prepared.

Tinctures

The alcohol-based extracts of plants, tinctures are much stronger than either teas or decoctions and so are taken in much smaller doses. For many plants alcohol is a better solvent than water because it can extract a wider range of plant constituents. It not only concentrates a remedy but also acts as a preservative. Stored correctly, a tincture will keep for up to three years.

Tinctures can be made from fresh or dried herbs, depending on the availability of the plants. When tinctures are manufactured, specific water-to-alcohol proportions are used for each herb, but for home preparation diluted vodka makes an excellent base.

Put 225 g (8 oz) of cut dried herb or 450 g (1 lb) of the fresh plant into a large jar. Pour 700 ml (3 cups) of vodka and 300 ml (1¼ cups) of water over the herb and close the jar tightly. Keep the container in a warm place for two weeks, shaking it well once a day. Strain the liquid through a muslin- or cheesecloth-lined strainer suspended over a bowl. Squeeze the remaining liquid from the residue into the bowl, then discard the solids.

Pour the tincture into a dark glass bottle and label with the name of the herb and the date prepared. It is now ready to use. Keep in a cool place away from direct sunlight.

A standard dose for a tincture is between 5 and 20 drops or up to 5 ml (1 teaspoon) three times a day for adults. Children under 12 should take 5 to 10 drops or up to 2.5 ml (½ teaspoon) three times a day. The tincture can be taken neat or mixed with a little water. Mixing drops of tincture with hot water will allow some of the alcohol to evaporate and leave just the herbal extract.

Syrups

Syrups are the traditional way of making medicines palatable for children. Sugar-based preparations also help to soothe and protect irritated and inflamed body tissue. The standard dosage for adults is 10 ml (2 teaspoons) three times a day; children should take 5 ml (1 teaspoon) three or four times a day, unless advised otherwise by a doctor or herbalist.

To make 1 liter (1 quart) of syrup, you need 225 g (8 oz) of dried herb or 450 g (1 lb) of fresh herbs, 2 liters (2 quarts) of filtered or bottled water, and 900 g (2 lb) of granulated sugar. Bring the water to a boil, then stir in the herb and simmer gently over low heat for 10 minutes. Strain the decoction through muslin or cheesecloth, taking care to squeeze all the liquid from the solid residue. Put the liquid in a clean pan and simmer over very low heat for about two hours or until reduced to 500 ml (2¼ cups). Add the sugar and stir over gentle heat until the sugar is completely dissolved. Be careful not to let the sugar boil or burn.

When the syrup is cool, pour it into a dark glass bottle, label, and store in a cool place. Syrups should be used within six months.

Capsules

Powdered herbs can be sprinkled on food or swallowed with water but are most easily taken as capsules. Capsule cases and powdered herbs are available from herb suppliers.

To prepare capsules, pour the powder into a saucer and slide the capsule halves through the powder. When they are full, join the halves together to seal the capsule.

Inhalants

Inhalants contain volatile oils and are used to relieve congestion and inflammation of the airways (see page 78). They are often added to hot water and the steam inhaled.

EXTERNAL PREPARATIONS

In preparations for external use, which include poultices, creams, and lotions, the active ingredients of an herb are incorporated into a form that can be applied directly to the affected area.

Essential, or volatile, oils are sometimes used instead of the herb itself. These are added to a base oil, cream, or wax, and they make preparation easier.

Compresses

Water-based herbal preparations that are applied directly to the skin with a cloth are called compresses. Because these can be prepared and applied quickly to the affected

Sage

Herb oils keep for months in a jar with an airtight lid.

Creams can be used liberally and will keep well.

Mallow and rose

Ointments are used on small areas only but can be stored.

Marigold

Lotions should be prepared fresh for each use.

Eyebright

Liniments are used sparingly, so a little goes a long way.

Cayenne pepper

Compresses are made by soaking a clean piece of cloth in a freshly prepared decoction or infusion.

Poultices are made to cover a specific area. You need only enough to repeat the treatment two or three times.

MAKING COMPRESSES AND POULTICES

Compresses can be applied hot or cold, depending on the condition for which they are used. Cold compresses are applied when the skin feels hot to the touch, in cases such as inflammation and swelling. Hot compresses are useful for relieving cramps and muscle tension. Poultices are used mainly to draw pus from the skin, heal abscesses and boils, and draw out splinters. You should prepare sufficient amounts of the herb to cover the affected area completely.

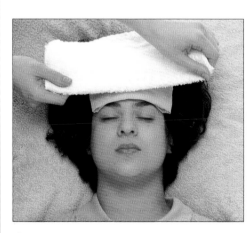

COMPRESSES
To make a compress, soak a clean cotton cloth in an herbal infusion or decoction, place it over the affected part, and cover with a clean towel. Continue to replace the compress to keep the area cool or hot as required. For cold compresses, make a slightly stronger infusion or decoction than usual and cool the liquid before use by adding ice cubes.

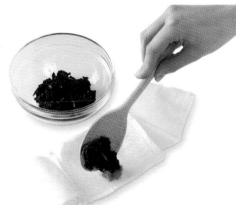

POULTICES
For a poultice, dried or powdered herbs are mixed to a paste with hot water and spread onto clean gauze before application to the skin. Rub some linseed or olive oil on the area to be covered, as this will make removal of the poultice easier. Cover with a cotton cloth and keep in place until the poultice has cooled. Repeat as necessary.

Making Your Own

Inhalants

Inhalants help relieve nasal congestion and fight sinus infections. You can rub them into the skin for inhalation over several hours or add them to hot water and breathe in the steam for immediate relief of symptoms. You can also inhale essential oils directly.

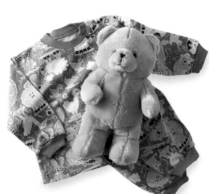

TODDLER TREATMENT
The discomfort of blocked airways is distressing to a child. This distress can be lessened with a few drops of essential oil on your child's bedding or teddy to help him or her settle into a comfortable night's sleep.

Essential oils like eucalyptus, pine, peppermint, and cajeput have long been known as effective decongestants and antiseptic remedies for illnesses that cause breathing problems, such as colds and hay fever. A selection of oils can be blended and inhaled directly by dabbing them onto a handkerchief or pillowcase. They can also be combined with a base of petroleum jelly and rubbed into the chest or added to hot water and the steam inhaled.

Because most essential oils are powerful, concentrated preparations, they should be taken only in very small quantities and used for the short-term relief of acute symptoms.

MAKING YOUR OWN VAPOR RUB

To prepare your own vapor rub, use a petroleum jelly like Vaseline as a base and add essential oils to it. When rubbed on the skin, petroleum jelly itself is not absorbed but allows the oils to evaporate slowly. Inhaling the vapors takes the oils' healing properties directly into the airways to soothe inflamed tissues and relieve congestion. Used sparingly, a vapor rub is suitable for infants and children. Stored in a cool, dark place, it will keep for up to a year.

Equipment
Small heatproof glass bowl
Wooden spoon or spatula
Small saucepan
Small glass measuring cup
Dark glass jar (50 ml/2 fl oz) or,
    two small dark glass jars
    (30 ml/1 fl oz) each
Labels

Ingredients
5 tbsp petroleum jelly
20 drops peppermint oil
20 drops eucalyptus oil
20 drops cajeput oil
5 drops pine oil

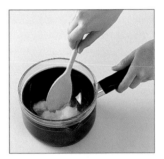

1 *Put the petroleum jelly in the bowl and suspend it over a saucepan that has been filled with enough water to cover the bottom. Heat slowly until the Vaseline has just melted.*

2 *Remove from the heat and transfer the petroleum jelly to the measuring cup. Cool for 2 minutes, stirring continuously.*

3 *Add the essential oils drop by drop, stirring continuously.*

4 *Pour the mixture into the jars. Leave to cool, then seal when the mixture has reached room temperature. Label each jar with the name and date.*

NIGHT-TIME RELIEF
Massaging vapor rub into your chest before you go to sleep will ensure that you inhale the decongestant vapors all night and awake breathing freely.

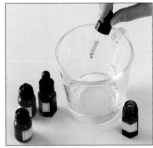

78

area, hot and cold compresses are ideal for relieving bruising, swelling, headaches, and many sports injuries.

Whether used hot or cold, for the best results compresses should be soaked and reapplied frequently.

Poultices

A warm paste of herbs applied directly to the skin and held in place with a dressing is called a poultice. The heat and active ingredients in a poultice make it ideal for infections and muscular pain. Traditionally, poultices were a favorite remedy for any type of skin infection.

Creams

Creams are light, nourishing preparations that spread easily and are absorbed into the skin. They contain natural waxes, oils, and a nonoily substance such as a tincture or a floral water. Creams are very useful for treating conditions that can affect large areas of the body, for example, dry skin, psoriasis, and eczema. Creams are particularly effective for treating conditions that need moisturizing, such as patches of rough, chapped skin. The cream forms a protective layer to reduce further complications, and the active herbal ingredients help to soothe the skin and heal the underlying disorder.

Ointments

Ointments are much thicker than creams because they consist of waxes and oils only, rather than a mixture of oil and water. They do not penetrate the skin very well, acting more as a protective barrier against infection and external factors. Use ointments for conditions that cover only a small area of skin, such as cuts, abrasions, and small patches of psoriasis. Underlying conditions that cause such skin problems may need other measures to combat the disorder, but ointments will help to relieve symptoms and speed recovery. If symptoms persist, seek

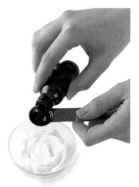

A SIMPLE CREAM
The easiest way to make an herbal cream is to add a tincture or essential oil to a base cream. Add 20 ml (4 tsp) of tincture or 8 drops of essential oil to 50 ml (2 oz) of unscented base cream (available from pharmacies).

MAKING CREAMS AND OINTMENTS

To prepare a cream from basic ingredients involves creating an emulsion between water and an oil or fat. The process must be carried out carefully to avoid separation. Once made, creams should be stored in airtight jars, preferably in the refrigerator, to keep them fresh. Unlike creams, ointments contain no water and are prepared with a base of petroleum jelly and beeswax or paraffin wax. The consistency of the ointment can be altered to suit the application—the more solid the ointment the less oily it will be.

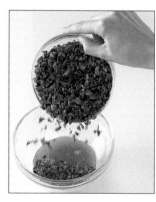

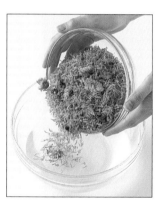

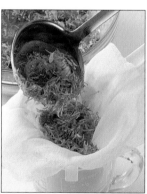

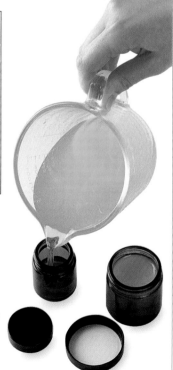

MAKING A CREAM
To make a cream, melt 175 g (7 oz) emulsifying wax (available from pharmacies) in a heatproof bowl over a pan of simmering water. Remove from the pan; stir in 25 g (1 oz) dried herb, 75 g (3 oz) glycerin and 75 ml (5 tsp) water. Return to the pan and simmer for 3 hours.

MAKING AN OINTMENT
Melt 450 g (1 lb) petroleum jelly or paraffin wax in a heatproof bowl over a pan of simmering water. Remove from the heat, then stir in 55 g (2 oz) finely chopped dried herb. Return to the pan and simmer for 15 minutes, stirring all the time.

1 *For both preparations, strain the hot mixture through a jelly bag or a strainer lined with muslin. Squeeze out excess liquid.*

2 *Cool slightly, then pour the still soft mixture into sterilized dark glass jars and leave to set. When cool, secure lids, label, and store.*

the advice of a qualified practitioner. It is possible that the action of the ointment may mask the signs of a more serious problem.

Liniments

Liniments are oily preparations designed to be easily absorbed through the skin to stimulate blood flow underneath. Very hot spices like cayenne pepper and mustard, for example, are traditional ingredients in a liniment. The skin will become very red and hot after application as the blood flow increases beneath the surface of the skin. This increased flow will help to heal an injury or infection.

MAKING LINIMENTS AND LOTIONS

Liniments are powerful healing tools for the pain of arthritic conditions and illnesses of the airways, but should never be used on broken skin because rubefacient herbs can irritate.

Floral waters like rose or chamomile water are good examples of skin lotions. They should be dabbed onto the skin with a clean cotton ball or pad or other absorbent fabric.

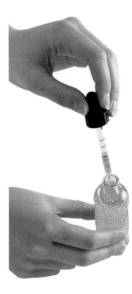

TO MAKE A LINIMENT
Mix one part of infused herb oil (see right) with an equal part of tincture; bottle and label it. For every 100 ml (3½ fl oz) of the mixture, you may add up to 10 drops of essential oils. A liniment will keep indefinitely and should be very well shaken before each use. Massage liniment gently into the skin and wash your hands afterward. Repeat as necessary.

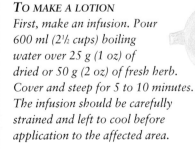

TO MAKE A LOTION
First, make an infusion. Pour 600 ml (2½ cups) boiling water over 25 g (1 oz) of dried or 50 g (2 oz) of fresh herb. Cover and steep for 5 to 10 minutes. The infusion should be carefully strained and left to cool before application to the affected area.

Larger, easily trapped pieces of fresh herb may not require straining.

Lotions

Lotions are liquid preparations for external use but unlike liniments, contain few or no oily substances. They can be applied directly to the skin as a compress or used as a wash for eyes, ears, or mouth. To make an eye lotion (see page 147), prepare a standard infusion, add a pinch of salt, and strain through a fine filter (coffee filters are ideal). Use with an eye-wash cup from a pharmacy or on a compress twice a day. Make a fresh infusion for each application and make sure the infusion is clear of any solids; you may exacerbate the problem if small pieces of herb get into your eyes. Use fresh lotion for each eye to avoid cross infection.

Infused herb oils

Unlike essential oils, infused herb oils are stable preparations and therefore do not evaporate, even when heated. Infused oils are particularly useful as massage oils and are important ingredients for many ointments, rubs, and liniments.

To make an infused oil, fill a clear glass jar with fresh herbs and cover them with a light vegetable oil—sunflower, grapeseed, or almond is suitable. Close the jar tightly and leave in a warm, sunny place for four to six weeks. Strain the oil through a sieve lined with cheesecloth or muslin into a large glass measuring cup, then pour it into a dark bottle, label, and date. Stored in a cool, dark place, it will keep for several months.

Other herbal preparations

In addition to the most common uses, many herbal remedies can be tailored to more specific treatments for various disorders.

Gargles and mouthwashes, for example, made from sage and thyme infusions are ideal for relieving sore throats and mouth ulcers. To obtain the best effects, use gargles as hot as possible .

Juices are simple to make and are easily applied externally or taken internally. A juice extractor, available from kitchen stores, makes juicing easy.

Plasters, cloth strips impregnated with wax and essential oils, are another way to apply herbs externally; as the body's heat softens the wax, the essential oils are released.

Pessaries and suppositories can also be made as herbal preparations. It is probably safest to buy ready-made pessaries and suppositories from an herbalist.

HERBS IN YOUR DIET

Many popular culinary herbs not only enhance the flavor of food but also have disinfecting and antioxidant properties that aid the digestive system in breaking it down.

Using herbs in food preparation is different from taking them medicinally; the amounts used for cooking are usually smaller. Nevertheless, even a touch of certain herbs in the diet may stimulate appetite, aid digestion, and help relieve gas.

USING HERBS FOR COOKING

A general rule of thumb is to use herbs and spices lightly at first, adding more as your taste dictates. Some—for example, bay, sage, celery seeds, rosemary, and thyme—can be particularly overwhelming or biting when used in large amounts.

Whenever possible, use fresh herbs; there are subtle overtones of flavor that cannot be duplicated with the dried versions. Herbs that are always much better in the fresh form include basil, parsley, and mint. When fresh herbs are not available, however, you can substitute dried ones by cutting the amount; the usual substitution is one part dried for three parts fresh.

You can also freeze herbs; most will retain their fresh color and much of their flavor, especially if blanched first. To blanch, dip a few sprigs at a time in a pot of boiling water; remove them, shake out the excess water, and dry them between towels. Put the herbs in plastic bags and seal and date them. Use them anytime for soups, salad dressings, stews, and sauces.

Heat releases the volatile oils in many herbs, and prolonged cooking can diminish not only flavor but also some of the healthful properties. To preserve their flavor and health benefits, add fresh herbs toward the end of a cooking period. Dried herbs generally hold up better in dishes that are cooked for a long time.

More herb flavor is released if you chop, bruise, or crumble the leaves before adding them to dishes. Herbs are also more flavorful served warm or at room temperature

HERBAL FEASTS
Many herbs make wonderful additions to salads and can be used in larger amounts than in other dishes. A salad of herbs is a delicious way to benefit from their therapeutic actions.

HERBAL TEAS

Culinary herbs need not be used only for cooking; they can also be the basis for a refreshing, soothing, invigorating, or calming cup of tea.

Culinary herbs that are particularly effective for making tea include thyme, mint, lemon balm, and fennel. Non-culinary herbs that make great tea are hops, rosehips, hibiscus, chamomile, lemon verbena, and meadowsweet.

For a refreshing and invigorating tea, use blackberry or blackcurrant leaves, rosemary, nettle, or peppermint. If you want a soothing and relaxing cup, after an exhausting day at work, for example, use aniseed, basil, fennel, or marjoram.

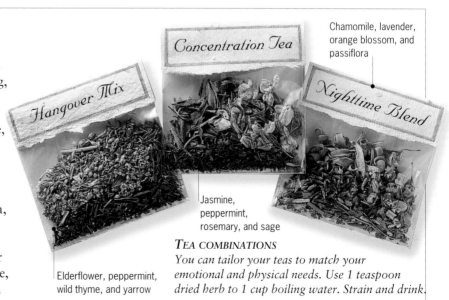

Chamomile, lavender, orange blossom, and passiflora

Jasmine, peppermint, rosemary, and sage

Elderflower, peppermint, wild thyme, and yarrow

Concentration Tea

Hangover Mix

Nighttime Blend

TEA COMBINATIONS
You can tailor your teas to match your emotional and physical needs. Use 1 teaspoon dried herb to 1 cup boiling water. Strain and drink.

HERBS AND SPICES FOR DIFFERENT DISHES

The following herbs and spices are all suitable for culinary purposes. Although many of them are recommended as complements for particular foods or types of dishes, there is no reason not to experiment by adding your favorites to any dishes you prepare. The difference between an herb and a spice is the part of the plant that is used. Leaves and flowers, used either fresh or dried, are considered to be herbs, whereas seeds, roots, and bark, usually dried and ground or their essence extracted, are deemed spices. Whether you are using fresh or dried products, the fresher they are, the better. All will lose intensity with age.

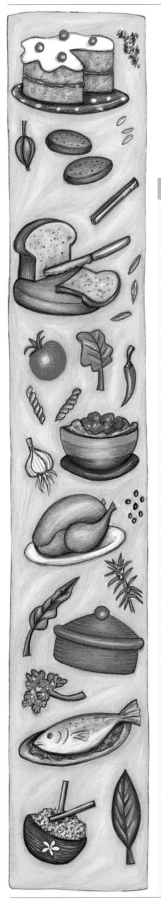

HERB/SPICE	CULINARY USE	THERAPEUTIC ACTION
Aniseed	Extract of seeds is used for flavoring cakes, cookies, and liqueurs; the leaves can be added to salads.	Acts as an appetite stimulant, helps to expel gas, and is a relaxing expectorant.
Angelica	The stems are often candied; the stalks can be cooked or eaten raw.	Aids digestion, relieves constipation, and freshens bad breath.
Basil	Along with garlic and tomatoes, the fresh leaves are basics in southern Italian cooking. Basil is also good in salads.	Clears the head and sinuses and helps to expel trapped gas.
Bay	One or two leaves are used to flavor soups and sauces, then removed.	Expels trapped gas.
Black pepper	The dried and ground seeds can be used to season almost any savory dish.	This aromatic digestive stimulant helps to expel trapped gas.
Caraway	The whole seeds are used to flavor breads, sausages, and coleslaw.	Caraway is calming to the digestive system and helps to expel trapped gas.
Cardamom	The ground seeds enhance sweet and savory dishes, especially in Indian cooking.	Expels trapped gas and relieves indigestion and headaches.
Cayenne pepper	The ground seeds are used sparingly to add fire to sauces and meat dishes.	Acts as a powerful digestive and circulatory stimulant; relieves stomach pains and cramps.
Celery seeds	These are used to enhance the flavor of soups, stews, and omelets.	They act as a digestive stimulant, help to expel trapped gas, and are a cleansing diuretic.
Cinnamon	The ground bark is popular in cakes, cookies, candies, and apple dishes.	Cinnamon is antiseptic and warming.
Coriander	The leaves (cilantro) are used in many Mexican dishes, ground seeds in curries.	Both the leaves and seeds are aromatic and disinfecting and help to expel trapped gas.
Dandelion	The leaves are cooked as a vegetable.	Dandelion is diuretic and cleansing.
Dill	Leaves are used in salads, sauces, and fish dishes, the seeds in making pickles.	Acts as an aromatic digestive stimulant and colic remedy; also helps expel trapped gas.
Garlic	Is a basic ingredient in sauces and many savory dishes, salad dressings, and dips.	Is anti-inflammatory and anti-infective, stimulates digestion, and promotes cardiovascular health.
Marjoram (also Oregano)	The leaves are favored in Italian dishes, salad dressings, stews, and stuffings.	Both are a warming digestive and circulatory stimulant.
Parsley	Leaves can be used in any savory dish.	Is disinfecting, cleansing, and diuretic.
Rosemary	The leaves can be used in salads or to flavor roasted meat or chicken; they also enhance potato dishes.	Is a warming digestive and circulatory stimulant; helps counter depression, fatigue, and rheumatic pains and enhance concentration and memory.
Sage	Leaves are used in poultry stuffings and stews of strong-flavored meats.	Is an antiseptic and digestive stimulant; helps relieve menopausal problems and diarrhea.
Thyme	Leaves are used to flavor meats, soups, cooked vegetables, and tomato sauces.	Acts as a disinfectant and expectorant; it also helps to relieve digestive problems.
Turmeric	The ground seeds are used in curries and fish and poultry dishes.	Turmeric is anti-inflammatory and soothing to the digestion.

CHAPTER 5

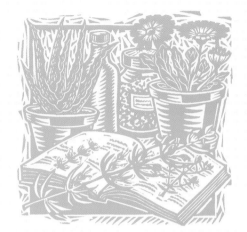

A GUIDE TO THE HEALING HERBS

To decide between a tincture of rosehips and a chamomile poultice, to find yarrow growing in the wild, or to know what to look for when harvesting goldenseal requires knowledge that has been refined over thousands of years. This chapter puts the knowledge at your fingertips and provides a valuable insight into the art of herbalism.

CHOOSING HERBAL REMEDIES

Knowing the active constituents of different herbs, as well as the various methods of preparation available, can give valuable insight to effective remedies for health problems.

Reading the recommended doses

On pages 86–133, all tinctures are noted as having a ratio—for example, 1:5—which means that for every 1 part of herb you should add 5 parts liquid. This liquid is always a mixture of water and alcohol, and the amount of alcohol is stated as a percentage, for example, 12%. Each recommended dose is given in milliliters.

All recipes for infusions are for weight in dried herbs; you should double the given amount if you are using fresh herbs. All the remedies should be taken three times a day, unless stated otherwise.

In this chapter you will find a selection of popular herbs and their recommended medicinal uses. For each herb there is a description of its physical characteristics plus an illustration, a guide to where it is commonly found, in some cases historical and background information, and the essential components of the plant. There is also a description of the actions of each herb, definitions of which are given in more detail on pages 52–55, and their best-known and most widely applied uses. This information is followed by recommended preparations and dosages. (Details about methods of preparation are given in Chapter 4.) Each entry concludes with any known cautions and contraindications.

CHEMICALS AND COMPOUNDS

The active constituents of an herb are the chemicals and compounds it contains that produce certain effects. The various constituents are grouped according to their active principles, or chemical makeup.

Herbs that are rich in alkaloids usually have strong pharmaceutical actions. An example is the capsaicin in chili peppers .

Anthraquinones are laxative. They stimulate the bowel after being absorbed into the system—hence their delayed action. Senna and rhubarb root contain anthraquinones.

Bitters are a varied group of constituents that have in common their bitter taste. The bitterness stimulates the salivary glands and digestive juices, which in turn improves appetite and digestion. Gentian and wormwood are bitters.

Coumarins are aromatic substances that are often used in perfumery. In the body they act as carminatives, antidepressants, and antiseptics. In pharmacology they are used as anticoagulants, that is, to help thin the blood. Herbs that contain coumarins include angelica and red clover.

Flavonoids also improve circulation by strengthening blood vessels and are often anti-inflammatory. Flavonoid-rich herbs include hawthorn and yarrow.

Mucilage and gums are viscous plant substances made up of molecules of complex sugars (polysaccharides). The sugar molecules soak up water to form a soft, jelly-like substance that coats the lining of the digestive tract with a soothing, sticky, protective layer. The soothing action extends to the lungs and bladder. Soothing herbs with a high mucilage content include fenugreek and marsh mallow.

Resins are liquids found in the stems of plants. With their antiseptic and antifungal actions, resins stimulate the immune system to fight infection. Echinacea and marigold are notable resinous herbs.

Tannins dry and contract the body's tissues, drawing them together and improving their resistance to infection. Herbs rich in tannins include tea and cinnamon.

Phenolic acids, although antiseptic and soothing when taken internally, can be very irritating when applied directly to the skin. Salicylic acid, the forerunner of aspirin, is one of the best-known phenols.

Antiarthritic herbs such as meadowsweet, contain soothing, analgesic salicylates. Aspirin was originally made from meadowsweet, but unlike aspirin, meadowsweet in its natural form does not upset the stomach.

The word *saponin* derives from *sapo*, which is Latin for soap. Like soap, saponins dissolve fats and can alter the balance of hormones in the body. Herbs rich in saponins include wild yam and ginseng.

LINNAEUS' HERBAL CLASSIFICATION

The herbs in this chapter are listed in alphabetical order under their Latin rather than their common names. The classification system using Latin names was originated by the Swedish botanist Carolus Linnaeus (Carl von Linné, 1707–1778) and has been used ever since as the most comprehensive and precise method of classifying plants. The Latin names will help you to be certain that you have exactly the right plant for your needs—not one that merely looks similar, is from the same family, or has the same or a similar common name. In many cases the difference can be crucial; neroli oil, for instance, comes only from the bitter orange plant, not from all orange plants, so accuracy is important. On the other hand, some plant genera, such as the aloes, all contain the same active ingredients. In these cases you will find the most common species listed.

COMMON NAME	LATIN NAME	COMMON NAME	LATIN NAME	COMMON NAME	LATIN NAME
Agrimony	Agrimonia eupatoria	Fennel	Foeniculum vulgare	Onion	Allium cepa
Aloe vera	Aloe vera	Fenugreek	Trigonella foenum-graecum	Oregon grape	Mahonia aquifolium
Angelica	Angelica archangelica	Feverfew	Tanacetum parthenium	Parsley	Petroselinum crispum
Apple	Malus spp.	Figwort	Scrophularia nodosa	Passionflower	Passiflora incarnata
Barley	Hordeum vulgare	Galangal	Alpinia officinarum	Peppermint	Mentha piperita
Basil	Ocimum basilicum	Garlic	Allium sativum	Plantain (psyllium)	Plantago spp.
Bay	Laurus nobilis	Gentian	Gentiana lutea	Pokeroot	Phytolacca americana
Betony	Stachys officinalis	Ginger	Zingiber officinale	Raspberry	Rubus idaeus
Bilberry	Vaccinium myrtillus	Goldenseal	Hydrastis canadensis	Red clover	Trifolium pratense
Bitter orange	Citrus aurantium	Hawthorn	Crataegus oxyacantha	Rose	Rosa spp.
Black haw	Viburnum prunifolium	Hops	Humulus lupulus	Rosemary	Rosmarinus officinalis
Bladderwrack	Fucus vesiculosus	Horse chestnut	Aesculus hippocastanum	Sage	Salvia officinalis
Borage	Borago officinalis	Horsetail	Equisetum arvense	Skullcap	Scutellaria lateriflora.
Burdock	Arctium lappa	Hyssop	Hyssopus officinalis	Sea holly	Eryngium maritimum
Chamomile	Chamomilla recutita	Juniper	Juniperus communis	Shepherd's purse	Capsella bursa-pastoris
Celery	Apium graveolens	Lady's mantle	Alchemilla vulgaris	St. John's wort	Hypericum perforatum
Chasteberry	Vitex agnus-castus	Lavender	Lavandula officinalis	Sweet flag	Acorus calamus
Chickweed	Stellaria media	Lemon	Citrus limon	Tea	Camellia sinensis
Chilies	Capsicum minimum	Lemon balm	Melissa officinalis	Thyme	Thymus vulgaris
Chinese rhubarb	Rheum palmatum	Linden	Tilia europea	Turmeric	Curcuma longa
Cinnamon	Cinnamomum verum	Licorice	Glycyrrhiza glabra	Valerian	Valeriana officinalis
Cleavers	Galium aparine	Lovage	Levisticum officinale	Vervain	Verbena officinalis
Coltsfoot	Tussilago farfara	Marigold	Calendula officinalis	Wild cabbage	Brassica oleracea
Comfrey	Symphytum officinale	Marsh mallow	Althea officinalis	Wild carrot	Daucus carota
Corn silk	Zea mays	Meadowsweet	Filipendula ulmaria	Wild yam	Dioscorea villosa
Cramp bark	Viburnum opulus	Motherwort	Leonurus cardiaca	Willow	Salix alba
Dandelion	Taraxacum officinale	Mugwort	Artemisia vulgaris	Wormwood	Artemisia absinthium
Echinacea	Echinacea angustifolia	Mullein	Verbascum thapsus	Yarrow	Achillea millefolium
Elder	Sambucus nigra	Nettle	Urtica dioica		
Elecampane	Inula helenium	Oats	Avena sativa		

Achillea millefolium YARROW

Yarrow is a member of the daisy family, which is native to Europe. It is widely distributed around pasturelands, meadows, and grassy roadsides, except in Mediterranean regions. It has now also colonized many of the English-speaking areas of the world, such as the United States, Canada, New Zealand, and Australia. Yarrow has finely divided leaves (*millefolium* means "a thousand leaves") and flat heads of tiny white, occasionally pink, flowers seen from June to September, when the herb is harvested. Since antiquity it has been a major herb in folk medicine throughout Europe. To gardeners, however, it is a troublesome weed, hard to eradicate because of its underground propagation. Yarrow's many active constituents include a light blue volatile oil (similar in many respects to chamomile oil), tannins, alkaloids, and a bitter principle.

Actions Yarrow has many traditional uses, yet it has never undergone extensive pharmacological investigation. Existing research, however, confirms its ability to reduce hemorrhaging, for example, and knowledge of many of its individual constituents supports most of its traditional uses. Some of yarrow's folk names—nose bleed, soldier's woundwort, sanguinary, and staunchweed—highlight its styptic, anti-inflammatory, and antibacterial properties. It is also antispasmodic, hypotensive, and diaphoretic, and helps to improve peripheral blood flow and warm the extremities—the hands and feet. These properties account for yarrow's long use as a tonic herb for circulatory problems of almost all kinds, including hypertension.

The volatile oil is responsible for several of yarrow's actions, being antispasmodic, carminative, anti-inflammatory and anthelmintic. Astringent and bitter properties added to its carminative actions make it an excellent digestive tonic. Like many antispasmodic herbs, yarrow is a uterine stimulant.

Uses As a circulatory herb, yarrow can aid hypertension, poor circulation, and varicose veins. It also has applications in a wide range of digestive problems, including poor appetite, sluggish digestion, gas and belching, inflammation of the digestive system (which should receive professional treatment), and bowel irritability. Infusions of yarrow are helpful in relieving colds and chills and recovery from infections. Taken regularly in small doses, yarrow helps to reduce excessive menstrual bleeding and cramps and to regulate the menstrual cycle.

Achillea millefolium

Dosage and preparations
Tincture – 1:5, 25%, 2–4 ml.
Infusion – 4 g per cup.

Cautions and contraindications
Avoid during pregnancy. A rare allergy to yarrow and some other herbs, such as chamomile, arnica, and marigold, causes temporary red pimply rashes. No other problems are known in normal use.

Acorus calamus SWEET FLAG

Also known as calamus, this vigorous marsh-loving plant with sword-shaped leaves is native to temperate and subtropical regions around the world. The North American variety was once used to relieve fevers, ease indigestion, and heal burns and boils, and was sometimes strewn over floors to sweeten the air in homes. The main active constituents are a volatile oil, a bitter principle, and tannins.

Actions Sweet flag stimulates the production of saliva and is a stomach tonic, increasing secretions and stimulating the appetite. Mildly sedative, it is traditionally used in Asia as a nerve tonic.

Uses An excellent digestive herb, sweet flag can be effective in easing heartburn, a poor appetite, poor digestion, and the feeling of bloatedness after meals. It relaxes the bowel and eases colic and flatulence. These actions, combined with sweet flag's mild sedative effect, make it useful in treating irritable bowel syndrome. The essential oil is very refreshing, especially for tired feet.

Dosage and preparations
Tincture – 1:5, 45%, 0.3–1 ml.
Infusion – 1 g per cup.

Cautions and contraindications
The Asian variety, now naturalized in North America, has caused tumors in laboratory animals. To avoid the risk of accidentally obtaining this variety, the FDA in 1968 declared all sweet flag (calamus) unsafe in the United States. In Canada, calamus products intended for internal use are not approved for sale.

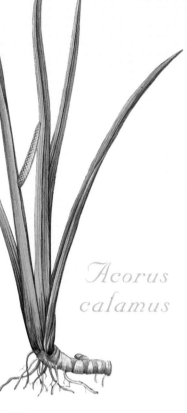

Acorus calamus

Aesculus hippocastanum HORSE CHESTNUT

The horse chestnut, a native of northern and central Asia, was probably introduced into North America in the late 18th century. This large, noble tree has leaf scars on its branches in the exact shape of horseshoes. Men once carried the seeds in their front pants pockets to ward off rheumatism, arthritis, and hemorrhoids. The seeds contain saponins, flavonoids, and tannins.

Actions Horse chestnut is an astringent tonic for the veins and capillaries, strengthening these vessels, improving blood flow, and decreasing swelling. It is mildly anti-inflammatory and diuretic.

Uses Horse chestnut is a good remedy when used externally as an ointment for conditions in which the veins are not functioning correctly, such as varicose veins, leg cramps, and hemorrhoids.

Dosage and preparations
Tincture – 1:5, 25%, 0.5–2 ml.
Ointment – add tincture to water-soluble base.

Cautions and contraindications
The nut is poisonous, and some herbalists recommend not using it in any form. In Germany, however, it is used to treat certain conditions under strict medical supervision. The leaves, flowers, and young sprouts are also toxic and should not be used in home remedies.

Aesculus hippocastanum

Agrimonia eupatoria AGRIMONY

A pretty, straight-stemmed plant, agrimony should be gathered from June, when the flowering yellow spikes appear, until the flowers die away. Agrimony contains a moderate quantity of tannins, which are drying and astringent, a little volatile oil, and a bitter principle.

Actions Agrimony combines bitter digestive tonic effects with a mildly astringent action, toning and healing the mucous membranes of the gut. It helps to regulate the function of the liver and gallbladder and it has been used in Germany to treat gallstones and cirrhosis. Historically, agrimony was greatly valued in wound-healing preparations. It was an ingredient in arquebusade water—named after the harquebus, an early type of gun—which was used to treat gunshot wounds in Europe in the 16th century. Chinese research has proved its efficacy as a blood clotting agent.

Uses The leaves are helpful for treating diarrhea or mild gastro-intestinal infections, especially in children. Agrimony is also one of the herbs of choice for an irritable bowel and colicky pains, especially when accompanied by loose bowel movements. An infusion is effective as a gargle for sore throats or a mouthwash for sore gums and mouth ulcers.

Dosage and preparations
Tincture – 1:5, 25%, 1–4 ml.
Infusion – 1–4 g, steeped for 10 minutes.

Cautions and contraindications
High doses may interfere with anti-coagulant and blood-pressure medicines. Agrimony may cause dermatitis after exposure to sun.

Agrimonia eupatoria

Alchemilla vulgaris LADY'S MANTLE

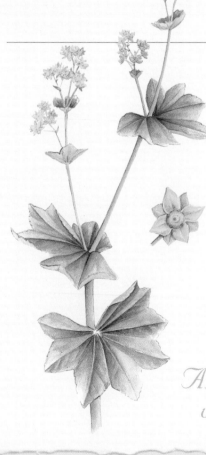

Lady's mantle grows across all of the northern hemisphere, including Europe, Asia, and North America. It is widely cultivated in private gardens for its soft, pretty foliage. The plant has an unusual reproductive cycle; the seed develops without fertilization from a male plant, a process known as parthenogenesis. The leaves and stems, which are collected between July and August, contain tannins and saponins.

Actions Lady's mantle has astringent and stomachic properties. It is often used as a digestive tonic and menstrual regulator and has a styptic action.

Uses Lady's mantle is a valuable herb for treating ailments of the female reproductive tract. It can be taken internally for irregular or excessive menstrual bleeding, for both of which professional advice should be sought, and for all menopausal symptoms. For external inflammation and itching, an infusion of the fresh leaves can be applied topically to the affected area. A strong infusion taken frequently is a good treatment for mild diarrhea, especially in children; it can also help to heal cuts and bruises when applied topically. For external applications, use either an infusion of the leaves or a decoction of the fresh root.

Alchemilla vulgaris

Dosage and preparations
Tincture – 1:5, 25%, or fresh, 1:2, 25%, 2–4 ml.
Infusion – 2 tsp per cup, infused for 10 minutes.

Cautions and contraindications
It should not be taken during pregnancy because of its styptic action.

Allium sativum GARLIC

Garlic cloves or corms (underground shoots) have been used medicinally, as well as in the kitchen, throughout known history. Grown all over the world, garlic contains a highly pungent volatile oil, minerals, and abundant antioxidants.

Actions Raw garlic is powerfully antibacterial and antifungal, especially one to three hours after crushing or bruising. Huge quantities of garlic were used during the First World War to disinfect wounds and prevent gangrene, just as they were by the Roman army over 2,000 years earlier. Garlic has often been used as a precaution during infectious epidemics. Raw garlic is also effective against intestinal parasites and helps to strengthen and protect the digestive tract. Garlic's antiseptic, volatile substances are excreted through, and disinfect, the lungs, skin, and urine, and thus the pungent odor is to some extent unavoidable.

Garlic has remarkable and well-researched positive effects on the heart and blood vessels, lowering blood pressure and cholesterol levels. It also adjusts the balance of fats in the blood, favoring those that inhibit clogging of the arteries (atherosclerosis). Garlic can help prevent the formation of clots in the blood vessels and break up those that have formed. In other words, it can be used to help reduce all of the major factors involved in degenerative heart disease.

Uses Garlic is used in the treatment of viral, bacterial, and fungal infections, whether internal or external, and has been proven very useful for relieving gastrointestinal infections. When applied externally, it can help to combat fungal infections such as vaginal candidiasis and athlete's foot, and help to clean infected wounds. Internally it is highly effective for keeping colds at bay. Garlic should be taken daily by anyone with a personal or family history of raised cholesterol levels, high blood pressure, or heart problems. Regular garlic intake is also beneficial for sluggish digestion and relieving gas and bloating, especially in older people.

Allium sativum

Dosage and preparations

To help clear up an infection of the digestive tract and prevent colds and flu, take one raw clove per day that has been bruised, chopped, or infused and left to cool. For acute infections, this quantity can be doubled. For problems of the circulation, take at least half a clove per day, dried, fresh, or in tablets or capsules. For external application, use a garlic infusion in a compress or cream.

Cautions and contraindications

Although generally very safe, garlic can irritate a sensitive digestive tract. Also, people who have clotting disorders or are taking anticoagulant drugs should not take medicinal amounts of garlic. Do not use raw garlic directly on the skin; it can cause burns. To reduce garlic breath, chew a sprig of parsley or eat an apple.

Allium cepa ONION

Onions have been cultivated for more than 6,000 years, and their medicinal benefits are widely applauded. They share many of the constituents of garlic, including antioxidants, minerals, flavonoids, and a volatile oil.

Actions As with garlic (see page 89), the expectorant, antibacterial, and antifungal properties of onion are most effective after crushing or bruising. Onions have a beneficial action on lipids in the blood, reducing the effects of dietary saturated fats and the buildup of fatty plaques. They also counteract rises in blood sugar, reduce blood clotting, and are believed to significantly reduce the risk of some cancers, especially that of the stomach.

Uses Onion is a very versatile household medicine. A small piece, lightly boiled, placed in the outer part of the ear can help to relieve the pain of earache, and fresh syrup of onion is an excellent disinfecting expectorant. A compress of roasted onion may help to relieve the discomfort of gout when placed on the painful joint.

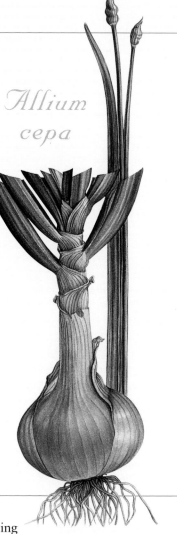

Allium cepa

Dosage and preparations
To achieve beneficial changes in blood lipids and the anti-infective effects, you need to eat at least half a strong raw onion every day. For other effects, cooked onions will suffice. A syrup can be made by putting equal amounts of sliced onion and sugar in a jar and draining off the resulting fluid a few hours later.

Cautions and contraindications
Raw onions may be overheating or excessively stimulating to some people, causing indigestion.

Aloe vera ALOE VERA

Aloe vera

A large succulent tropical plant that can easily be grown at home, aloe vera has a ring of spiny, fleshy, white-flecked leaves. The laxative juice from these leaves has long been used medicinally and is usually dried and sold as resin. The gel, exuded naturally when a leaf tip is cut, has antibiotic principles and has become a popular home remedy following its use as a healing agent during the Second World War.

Actions The bitter juice, or resin, is irritating to the bowel and has a cathartic action. The gel is a powerful healing agent, encouraging skin regeneration, yet is gentle enough to use directly on burns and wounds. It is also bacteriocidal and mildly laxative.

Uses Aloe vera gel is healing for mouth and skin ulcers, burns, wounds, dry skin, sunburn, and radiation burns. It also has a reputation, which is not yet adequately researched, for relieving gastrointestinal inflammation and calming an irritable bowel.

Dosage and preparations
Use the fresh gel or preparations rich in it, as required. There are high- and low-quality preparations available in health food stores and pharmacies.

Cautions and contraindications
Aloe resin is not recommended for home use, but it may be a component of proprietary laxatives. Do not take these for more than a week because they may lead to bowel flaccidity and mineral loss. Do not use them at all during pregnancy.

Alpinia officinarum GALANGAL

Galangal is a medium to tall east Asian perennial belonging to the same family as ginger. It has reedlike leaves and a cluster of white flowers. The rhizomes (root branches) have been used medicinally in Europe for more than 1,000 years and are known to have been used by Arabs to make their horses more fiery. The rhizomes smell pungent and spicy and have a taste similar to that of ginger. Galangal root contains volatile oil and resin.

Actions Galangal has properties similar to those of ginger but is gentler and less pungent. It is a diaphoretic, a circulatory stimulant, an aromatic digestive tonic, a carminative, and antibacterial.

Uses Galangal is mainly used for digestive problems, particularly bloating, colic, and gas after large meals. Like ginger, it can be used to prevent travel sickness and to quell other feelings of nausea. Its warming, diaphoretic effects make it a useful herb for fevers, though less stimulating than cinnamon, cayenne, or ginger. It is also used to relieve coughs and other cold symptoms.

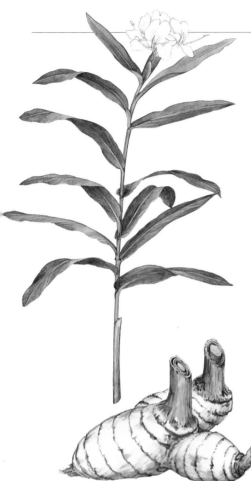

Dosage and preparations
Tincture – 1:5, 45%, 0.5–2 ml.
Infusion – 1–3 ml if powdered.
Decoction – 1 g per cup.

Cautions and contraindications
None are known.

Alpinia officinarum

Althea officinalis MARSH MALLOW

Marsh mallow is a perennial seashore-loving plant that grows in temperate regions worldwide. Its pink flowers grow on tall stems that are covered, like the leaves, with soft, velvety down. The leaves and roots contain mucilage, and the leaves and flowers contain a little volatile oil.

Actions The mucilage contained within the leaves and roots is a complex starch that absorbs water and becomes demulcent and emollient. The flowers and leaves are a soothing expectorant.

Uses Marsh mallow leaves and flowers are useful for dry, congested coughs and for cystitis. If boiled in distilled water, the leaves are also soothing for conjunctivitis. The infusion makes an excellent gargle and mouthwash for hoarseness, oral thrush, and gum abscesses. The root is primarily used for acid indigestion and diarrhea, although it also gives softness and bulk to stools and so may help to relieve constipation. When given to teething babies to chew, chunks of the peeled root help soothe the gums, and the dried root powder is a good drawing-out compound for splinters and boils.

Dosage and preparations
Tincture – 1:5, 25%, 2–4 ml.
Infusion – root: 1 part herb to 20 parts water, soak for 1–2 hours, then gently heat to 50°C (122°F) and leave to cool. Leaf/flower: 2 g per cup, infused for 10 minutes.

Cautions and contraindications
None are known, although excessive use may cause diarrhea.

Althea officinalis

Angelica archangelica ANGELICA

Angelica is an impressive plant that grows up to 2 m (6 ft 6 in) tall and is as widely grown for its appearance as for its candied stems, which are used to decorate cakes. It tastes and smells somewhat like juniper and was once used to dispel unpleasant smells in the home. The root, containing volatile oil, resin, and a bitter principle, is harvested at the end of the plant's first year in autumn or early spring. The leaves, also used occasionally, should be collected in June.

Actions Angelica is a warming circulatory stimulant, as well as being expectorant and antispasmodic. It is an excellent digestive tonic and is very useful in relieving loss of appetite and debility. It also has a long history of use as a general restorative.

Uses Angelica is one of the most widely used aromatic remedies and is helpful in convalescence as an appetite stimulant, for treating poor circulation, and for coughs. An infused oil of angelica and fennel is a good warming rub for a tight chest. The leaf has a gentler action than the root and is therefore more suited to treating children's ailments.

Dosage and preparations
Tincture – 1:5, 45%, 0.5–2 ml.

Cautions and contraindications
Angelica may encourage blood clotting and should be avoided by anyone with heart disease. Its use should be discontinued if it causes diarrhea or other problems.

Angelica archangelica

Apium graveolens CELERY

A popular salad vegetable, especially with dieters because of its very low calorie and high fiber content, celery is native to southern Europe but widely cultivated in Britain and North America. Its name, *graveolens*, means "strong smelling." The seeds, the main medicinal part of the herb, are used as a condiment and a salt substitute. They contain a volatile oil, coumarins, and flavonoids.

Actions Celery seeds have a mild diuretic and cleansing action and are believed to assist the elimination of uric acid, a buildup of which can lead to gout and kidney stones. They also have mild sedative properties.

Uses Celery seeds work particularly well alongside diuretics like dandelion leaf, and can be helpful in the treatment of arthritis and gout. They are also an aid to settling a sensitive digestive tract because they are mildly antispasmodic. The root, and to a lesser extent the stalks, share the actions of the seeds, and arthritis sufferers are advised to eat plenty of celery.

Dosage and preparations
Tincture – 1:3, 45%, 2–5 ml.
Infusion – 5 g per cup, or added to dandelion leaf infusion.

Cautions and contraindications
People suffering from kidney inflammation should avoid celery seeds.

Apium graveolens

Arctium lappa BURDOCK

A magnificent plant with large, soft, heart-shaped leaves and round heads of purple flowers, burdock grows on wastelands and along roadsides. The seed heads, covered with hooked spines that stick to fur and clothing, have inspired such names as cockle buttons and thorny burr. The sweet, mucilaginous root grows up to 1 m (3 ft) long and is harvested in the plant's first year. The burdock root contains a trace of volatile oil, and the seeds and leaves are also used medicinally.

Actions With its hypoglycemic, diaphoretic, and mildly diuretic actions, burdock appears to help move toxins from the tissues into the bloodstream to be removed by the kidneys and to some extent the skin and lungs. Burdock also has a bacteriostatic action.

Uses Burdock's main use is for skin problems such as acne, eczema, and psoriasis and for arthritis and other congestion-related conditions. To be fully effective, it should be taken over long periods of time, in small doses at first. The leaf and root are both used externally in soothing topical applications.

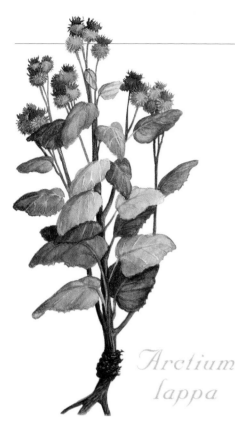

Arctium lappa

Dosage and preparations
Tincture – 1:5, 25%, 2–8 ml.
Decoction – 3 g per cup.
The fresh leaf juice, homemade or from health food stores, can be refrigerated or frozen.

Cautions and contraindications
Use in small doses at first to avoid overloading channels of toxin elimination, such as skin pores and kidneys.

Artemisia absinthium WORMWOOD
Artemisia vulgaris MUGWORT

Wormwood has gray-green hairy stems and feathery leaves. Mugwort produces clusters of small red or yellow flowers and dark green, deeply indented leaves. Both grow up to 1 m (3 ft) tall and are found along roadsides and other wastelands in temperate regions. Wormwood was once used in making the popular liqueur absinthe, outlawed in the early 20th century because of its hallucinogenic effects. Both herbs contain bitter glycosides, volatile oil, and tannins.

Actions Mugwort is a digestive tonic with a warming, aromatic, bitter action and has a slightly stimulating, restorative effect on nerves. It also eases uterine problems. Wormwood is a more bitter and powerful digestive stimulant that is anthelmintic.

Uses Mugwort helps regulate menstrual flow, aids digestive debility associated with fatigue, and is a natural insect repelant. Wormwood is used for poor digestion and loss of appetite associated with depression or convalescence. Traditionally it has been used to treat worm infestations and as an external antiseptic.

Dosage and preparations
Tinctures – both 1:5, 25%, 0.5–2 ml.
Infusions – mugwort 1–4 g, wormwood 1–2 g.
Wormwood can be used in the form of pills or capsules for worm infestations, but do not use more than 2 g, three times a day.

Cautions and contraindications
Avoid both herbs during pregnancy. Wormwood should be used only in small amounts and under a doctor's supervision. It has been declared unsafe in the United States by the FDA.

Artemisia absinthium

Artemisia vulgaris

Avena sativa OATS

Oats grow wild in temperate and cool climates and are widely cultivated all over the world as a food crop. The whole plant is used medicinally and is harvested when the seeds are developing in midsummer. Active ingredients include alkaloids, saponins, minerals, and B vitamins.

Actions Oat straw is a restorative that nourishes, sustains, and calms the nervous system while enhancing mood. Oat grains are very high in soluble fiber, which can help to soothe the digestive tract, improve bowel motility (to keep you regular), and lower cholesterol levels.

Uses Oats are good for convalescing from nervous debility, especially following such conditions as neuralgia and shingles. A useful alternative to stem preparations is oatmeal soaked overnight in water. This also makes a soothing application for dry and irritated skin and rashes caused by other plants.

Dosage and preparations
Tincture – (oat stems) 1:3, 25%, 1–2 ml doses as needed. Decoction – 20 g to 600 ml. Alternatively, 20 g oatmeal soaked overnight and taken in the morning.

Cautions and contraindications
Taken in large doses, oats can cause headaches. Oatmeal contains gluten, so gluten-sensitive people should avoid it, although a tincture or decoction should be gluten-free if left to settle, then separated from the sediment.

Avena sativa

Borago officinalis BORAGE

A rough, hairy perennial, borage has star-shaped blue flowers that attract bees and provide delicious honey. It is naturalized across Europe, and early settlers brought it to North America. The seeds contain gamma-linoleic acid, a fatty acid essential in nutrition. (The content is higher than that of evening primrose seeds.)

Actions The leaves and flowers of borage are diaphoretic, restorative, demulcent, galactagogue, and emollient. Dioscorides, a Roman army physician and author of the famous herbal *Materia Medica*, wrote that borage "cheers the heart and raises the spirits." Herbalists today use it to alleviate symptoms of stress and as a nerve restorative, an antidepressant, and to help support the adrenal production of hormones that regulate the body's systems.

Uses Traditionally, borage has been used to treat inflammation of the digestive tract, but has also found a place in the treatment of depression and nervous exhaustion. The hot infusion soothes a sore throat and induces sweating to ease fevers. As a poultice, borage soothes skin inflammations. The young leaves can be added to green salads.

Dosage and preparations
Tincture – 1:5, 25%, 1–2 ml.
Infusion – 2 g per cup.
Borage is best used fresh.

Cautions and contraindications
Borage contains alkaloids that, when taken in isolation, can cause liver damage. It is not recommended for prolonged internal use.

Borago officinalis

Calendula officinalis MARIGOLD

Marigold is a garden annual that ranges in height from 15 to 50 cm (6 to 20 in). It likes sunny locations and is native to the same regions as grapes, growing in vineyards, cultivated fields, and gardens. Double flowers from orange hybrids are preferred medicinally, as the ray florets—parts of the flowerhead that look like petals but are in reality each a tiny flower—contain the major medicinally valuable constituents.

Actions Marigold flowers are decongestant and astringent and help to heal tissue when applied topically. They have anti-inflammatory properties and are mildly diaphoretic and stimulating to the circulation. Their gum and resin contents are also antifungal, antibacterial, and antiprotozoan (protozoans are single-cell organisms, one type of which is responsible for malaria), but because these principles are not water soluble, preserving them requires a tincture very high in ethanol or an oil. A water-based extract has anti-inflammatory and antiviral properties and helps to boost the immune system.

Uses Whether taken orally or applied externally, marigold is an excellent treatment for recurring infections and chronic skin disorders. It is particularly useful (under professional guidance) in treating gastric infections and ulcers. The infusion also helps to bring on delayed menstrual periods and relieve menstrual pain.

A compress or a poultice using marigold is an excellent first-aid treatment for burns, scalds, stings, and impetigo—a highly contagious skin disorder—helping to soothe and heal. A cream or compress is also helpful for varicose veins, chilblains, and broken skin. A mouthwash or gargle is useful for mouth ulcers, gum disease, and throat infections.

An ointment or cream containing the tincture or infused oil, especially in combination with myrrh tincture or essential oil and tea tree essential oil, is an effective local treatment for fungal infections affecting the skin, nails, feet (athlete's foot, for example), or the vaginal area (such as candidiasis). A lotion made from an infusion also makes a useful compress for sore or inflamed eyes.

Calendula officinalis

Dosages and preparations
Tincture – 1:5, 25%, 0.5–2 ml.
Tincture to extract antibacterial gums and resins – 1:5, 90%, 0.5–1.5 ml.
Infusion – 1–2 g, infused for 5–10 minutes.
Infused oil – heat gently in sunflower oil.
A cream combining all of the therapeutic actions may be made by combining the water-based extract with oil or strong alcohol-based extracts.

Cautions and contraindications
Avoid during pregnancy because of its emmenagogue action.

Brassica oleracea WILD CABBAGE

Relatives of the cabbage that we commonly eat include herbs such as hedge mustard, black mustard, horseradish, and other vegetables of the crucifer family. Most share common constituents known as isothiocyanates, or mustard oil, the acrid, irritating basis of the mustard gas used during the First World War. Nonetheless, cabbage is medicinally useful in its natural state.

Actions Cabbage has two well-researched properties. First, cabbage-leaf juice has been found to be beneficial in healing peptic ulcers. Second, cabbage in any form is believed to play a role in the prevention of cancers, particularly colorectal cancers. It is thought that the cabbage's antimutagenic effect, which opposes and suppresses mutation, or abnormal changes, in the cells, derives from a natural defense against irritants. The bruised leaves, applied to the skin, are anti-inflammatory, anti-infective, and circulatory stimulants.

Uses The juice, taken in small, frequent doses over several weeks alongside other medications, is recommended for duodenal ulcers. A diet rich in cabbage and the other members of the crucifer family, such as Brussels sprouts and broccoli, is recommended for people with a family history of colon cancer. Applications of the bruised leaf are useful for both mastitis and hot, painful arthritic joints.

Brassica oleracea

Dosage and preparations
Fresh cabbage juice – 20–50 ml taken every few hours. Other preparations as above.

Cautions and contraindications
None are known.

Camellia sinensis TEA

Tea is a perennial evergreen that grows in tropical or subtropical areas. Archaeological evidence shows that tea was known 500,000 years ago, and as a beverage it is now second only to water in worldwide popularity. For black tea, commonly drunk in the West, the leaves are allowed to ferment after picking, whereas green tea, popular in the East, is brewed using unfermented leaves. Infusions contain polyphenols (tanninlike substances) and caffeine.

Actions Tea's paradoxical stimulating and calming effects on the nervous system are well known and are pharmacologically complex. Evidence from studies suggests a protective effect, especially from green tea, against cancers of the digestive tract, particularly the mouth, esophagus, stomach, pancreas, and colon. This may be due partly to its inactivation of carcinogens in cooked meat and fish and partly to its antioxidant effects. Drinking tea may also help to prevent strokes and fatty deposits in the arteries.

Uses Green tea drunk without milk may help to prevent cardiovascular problems and reduce the risk of some cancers. Black tea without milk is good for treating, as well as preventing, diarrhea.

Dosage and preparations
Tea can be drunk as an infusion, prepared to taste.

Cautions and contraindications
Large quantities of tea, especially taken without milk, may decrease absorption of nutrients, particularly iron.

Camellia sinensis

Chamomilla recutita CHAMOMILE

Chamomile grows on open ground in temperate regions. The flowers are distinguished from many similar-looking species by their hollow in the center. They are gathered between May and August and are best harvested as they begin to wilt; they should then be dried slowly. Their main constituents are a volatile oil and flavonoids.

Actions Chamomile calms the nervous and digestive systems and is also antispasmodic, mainly because of its water-soluble constituents. The essential oil is antiseptic, antifungal, and anti-inflammatory on mucous membranes and skin. Roman chamomile (*Chamaemelum nobile*) and German chamomile (*Matricaria chamomilla*) have similar properties.

Uses Infusions are good for easing tension, headaches, and irritability in adults and children, especially when associated with digestive problems, and they also help to relieve digestive problems associated with nervous tension and insomnia. Chamomile is especially good for irritable bowel syndrome and, in professional use, for inflammation of the digestive tract. Infusions also help to relieve menstrual cramps and sometimes migraines. Because of its anti-inflammatory properties, chamomile is particularly useful in the treatment of allergic conditions of the skin and upper respiratory system. A chamomile steam inhalation can help to ease sinusitis and asthma.

Chamomile is a versatile herb for external use because it reduces inflammation and promotes tissue healing. A cream or lotion helps to soothe inflammations of the skin, such as eczema, diaper rash, and cracked nipples, while a chamomile bath before bedtime relaxes the nerves.

Dosage and preparations
Tincture – 1:5, 45%, up to 5 ml.
Infusion – 5–8 g per cup, infused for 5 minutes with a lid on the vessel to retain the valuable essential oils. Loose chamomile generally seems to have a better flavor than teabags, perhaps because volatile constituents are lost when the flowers are shredded to make the latter. Essential oil – dilute to 10% in base oil or 20% in a cream. To make a chamomile bath, add 1 liter (1 quart) of a double-strength infusion to the bathwater, or run the hot water through a muslin or cheesecloth bag filled with chamomile flowers as you fill the bath.

Cautions and contraindications
In rare cases, it may cause an allergic rash. Large doses may bring on nausea.

Chamomilla recutita

Capsella bursa-pastoris SHEPHERD'S PURSE

Probably of European or western Asian origin, but now found worldwide except in the tropics, shepherd's purse is one of the most common and prolific weeds. The plant can grow as a single stem in a pavement crack or a bush on wasteland. The name refers to the plant's distinctive flat seed-pods. Shepherd's purse contains flavonoids and saponins.

Actions Shepherd's purse is styptic, astringent, and a urinary antiseptic. Its styptic action, confirmed by research, is mild, but its leaves were used to stanch bleeding during the First World War in the absence of ergot, a styptic fungus that grows on cereals and was used to treat wounds in the trenches. Shepherd's purse also causes the uterus to contract and is a mild circulatory stimulant. The herb also shows some anti-inflammatory, antiseptic, and antitumor potential.

Uses Traditionally, shepherd's purse was used for all forms of bleeding. It is now used mostly for heavy menstrual bleeding, and it should be combined with other herbs that address any hormonal cause of this problem.

Capsella bursa-pastoris

Dosage and preparations
Tincture – 1:5, 25%, 1–5 ml.
Infusion – 5 g per cup, steeped for 10 minutes.

Cautions and contraindications
Shepherd's purse should not be taken during pregnancy nor given to children under age two. The seed powder or tincture may irritate the skin.

Capsicum minimum CHILIES

There are several species and numerous varieties of chilies, or red pepper, the fiery fruits of a small upright tropical shrub. They include cayenne, anaheim, serrano, pasilla, poblano, and habanero. The popular sweet bell peppers also belong to the *Capsicum* genus, which is part of the nightshade family. The fiery-tasting alkaloid, capsaicin, gives red peppers their distinctive heat; they also contain beta carotene and vitamin C.

Actions A general stimulant, chili pepper is also a digestive and circulatory tonic, an anticoagulant, an antispasmodic, and an analgesic. It is expectorant and decongestant and thins secretions, such as phlegm and mucus. The red pepper's remarkable range of actions are associated with its powerful heating and stimulating properties.

Uses Chili stimulates the appetite and is useful for sluggish digestion, colic, and flatulence. It is a heating circulatory stimulant, helping to stave off a chill or the start of a cold. Used externally, it produces redness and warmth, relieving stiff joints and nerve or muscle pain.

Capsicum minimum

Dosage and preparations
Tincture – 1:10, 60%, 0.3–1ml, well diluted.
Powder – 30–50 mg.
The powder can be infused in oil or added to a cream for external application.

Cautions and contraindications
It is not recommended for sufferers of hypertension or gastric irritation except under professional supervision. Do not ingest *Capsicum* tinctures and alcoholic extracts. Avoid contact with eyes and other mucous membranes.

Cinnamomum verum CINNAMON

Cinnamon, derived from the inner bark of a tropical tree, is native to several tropical climates, including Sri Lanka, southeastern India, and Central and South America. It is one of the world's oldest folk medicines. The main constituents are a volatile oil, coumarins, and tannins.

Actions Cinnamon is a warming digestive and a circulatory stimulant. It is antispasmodic and a carminative with an antidiarrheal effect, and it acts to improve the action of the stomach and digestive secretions. It is also a powerful antiseptic.

Uses Cinnamon is effective for poor appetite, especially when associated with sluggish digestion and a feeling of coldness. The warming effect is useful in treating chesty colds (especially when mixed with ginger) and influenza (when mixed with elderflower and peppermint). A cinnamon infusion improves circulation to cold hands and feet and is a good general tonic in prolonged illness. Cinnamon is also used for treating inflammation of the mouth and pharynx. Chinese cinnamon *(Cinnamomum aromaticum)*, also known as cassia, is used in Chinese medicine to treat impotence and rheumatic conditions.

Cinnamonum verum

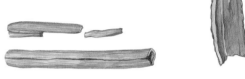

Dosage and preparations
Tincture – 1:5, 45%, 0.3–1 ml. Infusion – 0.5–1 g, taken as necessary for colds and flu.

Cautions and contraindications
Do not use medicinal quantities during pregnancy as it may cause miscarriage. Cinnamon oil taken internally can cause nausea, vomiting, and kidney damage.

Citrus aurantium BITTER ORANGE

A native of tropical Asia, the bitter orange tree is now widely grown in all Mediterranean countries. The fruits are rich in vitamin C and contain flavonoids in the peel.

Actions Consumption of any citrus fruit can help to protect against cancer of the stomach, esophagus, and possibly of the pancreas. The juice is effective against some viruses, and the pectin in the skin and membranes of both oranges and grapefruit has been found to help lower blood cholesterol.

Uses Infusions of bitter orange peel and orange flowers are good for insomnia. Dried bitter orange peel was once used as a digestive tonic in the West and continues to ge given as a warming stomachic in Chinese medicine. Bitter orange flowers yield a fragrant and expensive volatile oil—neroli—which is used in high-quality perfumes and aromatherapy. An infusion of the flowers is also useful.

Citrus aurantium

Dosage and preparations
For the full cardiovascular benefits of oranges, eat the pithy parts and the membranes, as well as the flesh, and add the zest to orange juice. The vitamin C is quickly lost to the air, so drink the juice as soon as possible after pouring. Infusion – (orange flower or peel) 2–3 g per cup, steeped for 5 minutes.

Cautions and contraindications
This fruit may aggravate inflammatory conditions in some people and hyperactivity in children.

Citrus limon LEMON

Renowned throughout the ages as a health-giving fruit, the lemon is rich in vitamin C. One of the most famous medicinal uses of citrus came about through an old British navy regulation that stipulated an ounce of lemon or lime juice a day for every sailor after 10 days at sea to prevent scurvy—hence the nickname "limeys."

Actions Lemon juice is disinfecting, antiviral, expectorant, and astringent. The peel and pith are high in bioflavonoids; they are also thought to be anticarcinogenic and capable, in large amounts, of lowering blood cholesterol. Lemon yields a volatile oil that is being investigated for use as a therapy for certain types of cancer

Uses The juice with water is an excellent gargle for sore throats. Honey and lemon infusions are disinfecting and mildly expectorant for colds and fevers. The oil is effective topically for viral warts. Citric acid works safely as a gastric stimulant, digestive bitter, mild antiseptic, and topical exfoliant.

Dosage and preparations
Infusion – 2 slices per cup for colds, combined with honey and ginger or cinnamon. Essential oil – use directly on the wart but avoid contact with surrounding skin.
To gargle, dilute the juice of half a lemon in a wine glass of warm water.

Cautions and contraindications
Lemon juice erodes tooth enamel, so rinse your teeth with water after contact. Excessive consumption of lemon can cause irritation of the esophagus and stomach.

Crataegus oxyacantha HAWTHORN

Also known as mayflower (for which the Pilgrims' famous ship was named), hawthorn was brought to North America by English settlers, who used it in teas and tinctures for stomach and bladder problems. The species hybridizes freely, and the leaves, flowering tops, and berries all have similar properties. The leaves in particular are rich in glycosides and tannins.

Actions The properties of some of hawthorn's active constituents are well understood and present a remarkable picture of what herbalists refer to as synergy—meaning "working together." Some constituents strengthen the heart's action; others slow it slightly and improve its blood supply. The net effect is to make a weak heart work more efficiently and to reduce blood pressure. Hawthorn must be used long-term to have any significant effect.

Uses A good herb to take daily—along with garlic—by anyone over 40 years old with a history of hypertension or heart disease in the family. As a supplement to other therapies, it is helpful for most degenerative conditions of the heart or blood vessels

Dosage and preparations
Tincture – 1:5, 25%, 1–2 ml.
Infusion – 5 g of flowers and leaves per cup.

Cautions and contraindications
No known side effects, but if you are taking medicine for arrhythmias or heart failure, especially digoxin, use hawthorn only under professional supervision.

Crataegus oxyacantha

Curcuma longa TURMERIC

Native to southern Asia, turmeric is a member of the same family as ginger and is an important spice in curries and other Indian food. It contains a volatile oil, vitamins, minerals, and the pigment curcumin, which is a common yellow-orange coloring agent for food.

Actions The alkaloid curcumin in turmeric produces anticlotting, anti-inflammatory, and antioxidant effects. Turmeric is also carminative (soothing to the digestion) and cholagogue (restorative to the liver).

Uses Turmeric is a valuable herb in treating gallbladder and liver problems and helpful in poor digestion associated with chronic fatigue and inflammation. It has proven anti-inflammatory effects that are very helpful in relieving the pain of rheumatoid arthritis. As an antioxidant, turmeric is recommended for degenerative circulatory disorders, and it shares many uses with its relation, ginger, such as improving circulation, calming inflammation, and detoxifying the body. It is used in China for shoulder pain and menstrual cramps and in India for liver disease.

Dosage and preparations
Powdered herb – 1–3 g per day, mixed into a thick liquid, such as apple or pear concentrate, or made into pills with honey.

Cautions and contraindications
Do not give to children under age two. People with gallstones or ulcers should use turmeric only after consulting a doctor. Topical use may cause a rash.

Daucus carota WILD CARROT

Commonly known as Queen Anne's lace, wild carrot grows across most of temperate North America. It is the same species as cultivated carrot, but the root is pale in color, acrid to the taste, and very aromatic. Its leaves and seeds contain a volatile oil and an alkaloid; the roots of both varieties are rich in bioflavonoids, including beta carotene.

Actions The roots of both wild and cultivated carrots are soothing to the digestive system and seem to be powerfully protective against some cancers, notably those of the lung, colon, and pancreas, probably because of the bioflavonoids. Wild carrot seeds and, to a lesser extent, the aerial parts of the plant (leaves, stalk, and flowers), are carminative, antiseptic, and diuretic.

Uses Carrots are a valuable food, particularly suited to people with sensitive digestive systems; when eaten two or three times a week, they can help improve night vision. Two or more carrots a day may give significant protection against many forms of cancer. Infusions or tinctures of the seeds, together with frequent drinks of water, ease flatulence and are useful for treating cystitis or prostatitis. Carrot tea is mildly anthelmintic.

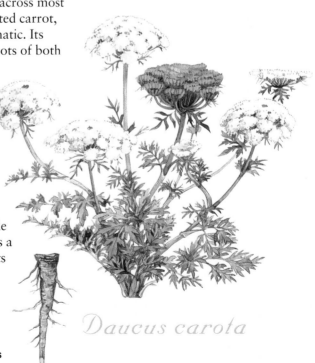

Dosage and preparations
Tincture – (herb and seed) 1:5, 45%, 1–2 ml.
Infusion – (herb and seed) 1–2 g per cup, steeped for 10 minutes.

Cautions and contraindications
Do not take carrot seeds during pregnancy.

Dioscorea villosa WILD YAM

Wild yam, as the name suggests, is the wild relative of the edible yam, a native of Mexico and the southern United States. It has a densely matted rootstock, which contains steroidal saponins, alkaloids, tannins, and starch.

Actions Wild yam is anti-inflammatory, antirheumatic, and antispasmodic. It also has the effect of being diaphoretic and cholagogue. Its anti-inflammatory action may be due to the steroidal saponins. These have been used as a raw material for the production of the progesterone-only contraceptive pill, and although they are not converted in the body to progesterone, they are likely to have an influence on steroid hormone function.

Uses Wild yam is useful for relieving inflammation and colicky conditions of the digestive tract, such as irritable bowel syndrome, stomach cramps, and inflammatory bowel disease (only under professional guidance). It is also a major anti-inflammatory herb and is helpful in easing such conditions as rheumatoid arthritis. In recent years it has been seen more as a hormonal tonic, and it is useful for weakened hormonal production, menstrual pain, and menopausal problems, particularly cramps and lack of energy.

Dosage and preparations
Tincture – 1:5, 45%, 2–10 ml.
Decoction – 1 tsp per cup, simmered for 20 minutes.

Cautions and contraindications
Avoid during pregnancy because of the effect on hormone production.

Dioscorea villosa

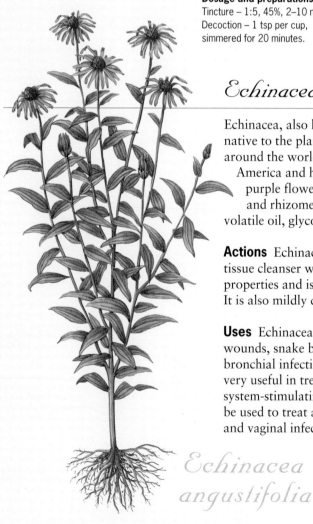

Echinacea angustifolia ECHINACEA

Echinacea, also known as purple coneflower, has three major species, all native to the plains of central North America, though they are now cultivated around the world. *Echinacea purpurea* has the widest distribution in North America and has been extensively studied. With distinctive, large-petaled purple flowers, echinacea can reach up to 2 m (6 ft) in height. The root and rhizome, and occasionally aerial parts, are used and contain a volatile oil, glycosides, polysaccharides, and a resin.

Actions Echinacea is a well-researched immune stimulant and a powerful tissue cleanser with vulnerary properties. It has antibacterial and antiviral properties and is particularly effective against herpes and influenza viruses. It is also mildly diaphoretic.

Uses Echinacea was a major medicine for Native Americans, used for wounds, snake bites, and fevers. It is excellent for ear, nose, throat, and bronchial infections, especially those that are prolonged. It has been found very useful in treating colds and flu because of its mild diaphoretic, immune-system-stimulating, and antiviral actions. As a tissue cleanser, echinacea can be used to treat abscesses; applied externally to skin ulcers, infected wounds, and vaginal infections; and taken as a gargle for throat infections.

Echinacea angustifolia

Dosage and preparations
Tincture – 1:5, 45%, 1–3 ml.
Infusion – 1–2 g per cup, infused for 10 minutes.

Cautions and contraindications
None are known, yet the herb is not recommended for pregnant and nursing women, diabetics, children under two, or people with serious illnesses.

Equisetum arvense HORSETAIL

Horsetails are a primitive, nonflowering group of plants that reproduce by releasing spores. Their giant ancestors, along with ferns, once covered the planet, and their fossils form our coal seams. Horsetail grows on wasteland, often above underground streams. The long, green, sterile stems of summer, rather than the brownish fertile stems seen in spring, make the best harvest. They contain flavonoids and minerals. Correct identification is crucial because horsetail's relative, *E. palustre,* contains a toxic alkaloid.

Actions With anti-inflammatory and astringent actions in the genitourinary tract, horsetail is also mildly diuretic. It aids blood clotting and is used to heal connective tissue, particularly in damaged lungs and arthritic joints.

Uses Useful in treating mild cystitis and bed-wetting, horsetail has a long history of use for rheumatic conditions and may help to repair sprains, fractures, and weak or brittle nails. Externally, it is a useful styptic and healing agent for wounds.

Dosage and preparations
Decoction – to draw out the active ingredients, grind and boil the herb for several hours. Use 25 g of horsetail per 600 ml of water, with a little sugar.

Cautions and contraindications
It is inadvisable for people who have edema due to heart or kidney disease to use horsetail.

Equisetum arvense

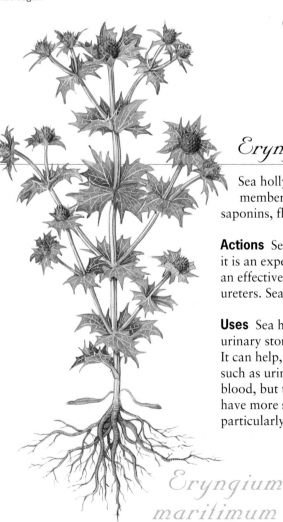

Eryngium maritimum

Eryngium maritimum SEA HOLLY

Sea holly, common on the sandy shores of northern Europe, is a member of the carrot family but looks more like a thistle. It contains saponins, flavonoids, and the aromatic substance coumarin.

Actions Sea holly root shares many of the properties of angelica root, in that it is an expectorant, a diaphoretic, and a nervous system restorative. It is also an effective, relaxing diuretic that increases urinary output and relaxes the ureters. Sea holly was once very popular candied, although this is now rare.

Uses Sea holly has traditionally been used to relieve renal colic and to clear urinary stones. It is also helpful for easing the pain of cystitis and prostatitis. It can help, especially in combination with horsetail, to relieve symptoms such as urinary frequency, irritation, and the passing of small amounts of blood, but these symptoms need professional evaluation because they can have more serious implications. Sea holly can also be used to relieve coughs, particularly whooping cough.

Dosage and preparations
Tincture – 1:5, 25%, 5–8 ml.
Infusion – 1 tsp of shredded root per cup, steeped for 10 minutes.

Cautions and contraindications
The appearance of blood in the urine always requires professional investigation.

Filipendula ulmaria MEADOWSWEET

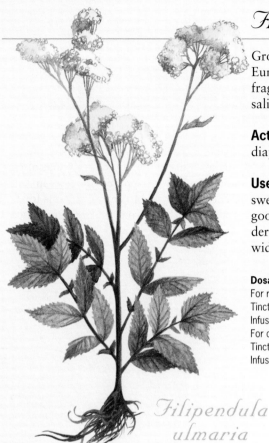

Growing in abundance on banks and ditches across North America, Europe, and temperate Asia, meadowsweet produces tufts of small, fragrant, creamy-white flowers. The flowering herb contains tannins, salicylates, and a volatile oil.

Actions Meadowsweet is anti-inflammatory, antiseptic, antipyretic, and diaphoretic. When used topically, it is also rubefacient and analgesic.

Uses Meadowsweet has long been used for urinary infections, to induce sweating in high fevers, and for infantile diarrhea. It is a stomachic herb, good for acid indigestion and heartburn—in contrast to aspirin, which derives from it but can irritate the stomach lining. Meadowsweet is widely used as an anti-inflammatory herb for arthritis and rheumatism.

Dosage and preparations
For rheumatic conditions large doses are needed:
Tincture – 1:1, 25%, 5 ml.
Infusion – a daily dose of 50 g.
For other conditions:
Tincture – 1:5, 25%, 1–2 ml.
Infusion – 1 g per cup, steeped for 5 minutes.

Cautions and contraindications
Do not use in conjunction with anticoagulant therapy or anti-inflammatory drugs. Pregnant and nursing women and people allergic to aspirin should not take the herb; children should be given it only with medical supervision.

Filipendula ulmaria

Foeniculum vulgare FENNEL

This erect biennial thrives on dry soils in Mediterranean and other temperate regions, producing umbrella-type spokes of yellow flowers from July to October. The threadlike leaves are much used as a condiment, especially with fish, and the root is an aromatic salad vegetable. The seeds are used medicinally and as a condiment and digestive. They contain a volatile oil that includes anethole, also found in aniseed, and some related compounds with estrogenic properties that act like the female hormone estrogen.

Actions Relaxing and warming to the digestive system, fennel is also a mild antidepressant and a gentle bronchodilator that relieves asthma. Anethole is structurally similar to some of the major mood-regulating neurotransmitters in the brain. It is galactagogue and emmenagogue. The medieval herbalist Hildegarde of Bingen regarded fennel as an all-purpose herb that promoted good health.

Uses The seeds relieve indigestion, infant colic, and flatulence. They are also a gentle expectorant, mainly used for children. Fennel is excellent for nursing mothers, increasing the flow of breast milk, and because the volatile substances are passed through the breast milk, it helps to relieve colic in babies.

Dosage and preparations
Tincture – 1:5, 45%, 1–2 ml.
Infusion – 2–4 g of seeds per cup.

Cautions and contraindications
Do not take high doses for long periods. Never ingest pure fennel oil. Do not use if you are pregnant or have liver disease.

Foeniculum vulgare

Fucus vesiculosus BLADDERWRACK

The thallus, or frond, of this common seaweed, also known as kelp, is gathered in early to midsummer and then dried rapidly. It contains minerals, most notably iodine, a wide range of trace elements, including chromium, and polysaccharides (mucilage).

Actions Kelp has been used since the 18th century to treat goiter, a swollen, underactive thyroid gland, because the thyroid requires iodine to make its hormone, thyroxine. It has also been used—although not clinically proven to help—in treating obesity. There are probably several reasons for this. Kelp helps stimulate the thyroid, while the presence of chromium helps to prevent the accumulation of fat.

Uses Possibly helpful in treating obesity and thyroid underactivity (under professional supervision), bladderwrack is also used as a bulking agent to relieve colic and constipation and as a traditional remedy for arthritic stiffness and pain.

Dosage and preparations
Take up to 2 g of dried herb or fresh equivalent daily in a tea, tincture, decoction, or as tablets.

Cautions and contraindications
Weight loss with the aid of herbs should be attempted only under professional supervision. Excessive amounts may overstimulate the thyroid gland, putting a strain on the heart.

Fucus vesiculosus

Galium aparine CLEAVERS

An angular, rough and hairy plant, cleavers has leaves in whorls (rings around the stem) and tiny flowers that are followed by hairy fruit. The fruit adheres to clothing, fur, or hair, giving rise to the old common names of catchweed, stick-back, and sticky jack. The roasted seeds can be used as a coffee substitute. The aerial parts are gathered in May and June, when coming into flower, and contain glycosides, phenolic acids, and tannins.

Actions A mild diuretic, cleavers is believed to relax the urinary vessels, facilitate the passage of small urinary stones, and help dissolve calcium stones. Cleavers is one of the main remedies for stimulating the lymphatic system, which drains excess fluid and toxins from the body's tissues.

Uses As a tissue cleanser, cleavers is commonly used for skin diseases, particularly psoriasis, as well as conditions in which the lymph glands are enlarged. It can be used to drain excess fluid and is a traditional slimming aid. Cleavers was once used to dissolve or expel kidney stones. The roots were also dried and powdered and put on wounds to promote healing.

Dosage and preparations
Preparations made from the fresh herb are best.
Tincture – 1:5, 25%, 5–10 ml.
Juice – 5–10 ml, refrigerated or made into ice cubes.

Cautions and contraindications
It is safe in normal use; there are no known contraindications.

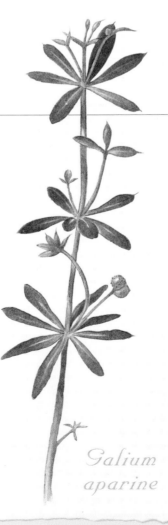

Galium aparine

105

Gentiana lutea GENTIAN

Native to mountain regions in central and southern Europe and western Asia, gentian is an attractive medium to tall perennial that produces clusters of golden flowers in the upper leaf axils. The root and rhizomes are the main parts used. The root tastes sweet at first, then intensely bitter, because of the presence of bitter glycosides.

Actions A bitter digestive stimulant and anti-inflammatory, the bitter principle increases saliva production and stimulates the appetite and the digestive juices. Gentian is an important ingredient in some aperitifs, taken before a meal to improve appetite and digestion. The bitterness can be tasted at extremely low concentrations, so gentian should be used sparingly to avoid irritation and unpleasant aftertaste.

Uses Gentian is used specifically for stimulating appetite and improving sluggish digestion and elimination. It has also been used to relieve stomachache, heartburn, and nausea.

Dosage and preparations
Tincture – 1:5, 25%, 10–20 drops an hour before meals. Infusion – 0.5–1 g.

Cautions and contraindications
Some people are very sensitive to bitters, and gentian may give them headaches. Gentian is inadvisable for sufferers of stomach and duodenal ulcers.

Gentiana lutea

Glycyrrhiza glabra LICORICE

Glycyrrhiza glabra

Licorice likes sandy soil and has lived for thousands of years in the floodplains of southeastern Europe and southwest Asia. The root and stolons (runners) have been used medicinally for at least 3,000 years. They contain glycosides, mucilage, and intensely sweet saponins (*glycyrrhiza* means "sweet root").

Actions Licorice forms a soothing coating in the stomach and other parts of the digestive tract, which encourages mucus production. It also acts as a soothing expectorant for coughs. Antispasmodic and healing, licorice's saponins, similar to the body's own steroid hormones, increase some hormonal effects. They counteract inflammation and promote water and sodium retention. Licorice root is also antiviral, notably against the herpes simplex (cold sore) virus.

Uses Licorice is effective as an expectorant and cough suppressant. It is commonly used in prescriptions for arthritis, eczema, asthma, mouth ulcers, heartburn, gastritis, and peptic ulcers (drugs have been developed from it for treating ulcers). It is often used (professionally only) for supporting steroid withdrawal and poor hormone production. Externally, it is helpful for cold sores and eczema.

Dosage and preparations
Tincture – 1:3, 25%, 1–2 ml. Decoction – 1 tbsp per 600 ml, simmered for 20 minutes, or chew the dried root.

Cautions and contraindications
Used for more than six weeks, it can cause edema and potassium loss. People with cardiovascular disease, high blood pressure, or liver or kidney problems should use only with medical supervision.

Hordeum vulgare BARLEY

Barley has been grown as a food crop in the Northern Hemisphere for at least 6,000 years. Roman gladiators ate it to build up their physical strength, and it is a staple across the world. It is a well-balanced food, high in starch, lysine, fiber, calcium, iron, magnesium, and potassium.

Actions   Extensive research by the Department of Agriculture in the United States has established barley's action to reduce levels of low-density lipoproteins (LDLs) in the blood. The substances responsible are found mainly in the bran, but also throughout the kernel. Green barley, the juice of young barley leaves, is a concentrated source of vitamins and minerals and is high in superoxide dismutase (SOD), a potent antioxidant that is thought to reduce many of the effects of aging.

Uses   A grain commonly used in bread, flour, soups, stews, and sauces, barley helps to prevent heart and circulatory diseases. Green barley is a useful nutritional supplement for preventing or remedying nutritional deficiencies, especially those of iron, magnesium, and potassium. It is also an antioxidant with cardio-protective and possibly cancer-preventing properties. Barley and barley malt are nourishing for convalescents. Barley drinks are soothing to intestinal disturbances and inflammatory bowel irritations.

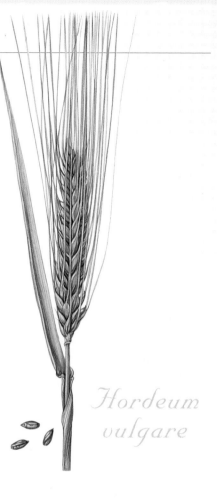

Hordeum vulgare

Dosage and preparations
Green barley – a glass of the fresh juice morning and night.

Cautions and contraindications
Do not take if you have gluten sensitivity.

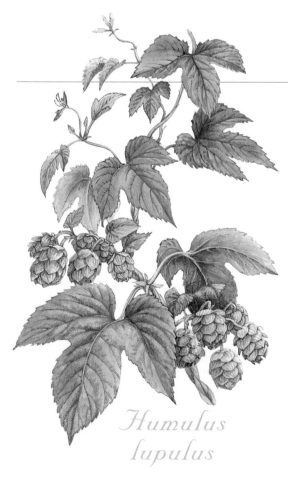

Humulus lupulus

Humulus lupulus HOPS

A tall, climbing perennial that grows around riverbanks, hops have been cultivated since Greek and Roman times. The clusters of female flowers, used for brewing beer as well as for making medicines, contain a bitter resin, a volatile oil, flavonoids, and an estrogenic substance. Hops give beer its slightly bitter flavor and help preserve it.

Actions   Many compounds in hops contribute to a sedative action. The bitter resins are strongly antibacterial and anti-inflammatory but degrade fairly quickly in the dried plant, producing a volatile substance that is also sedative.

Uses   Reduces irritability and restlessness, especially with insomnia; because of its sedative effect, it is also effective in relieving anxiety. Hops are good for improving appetite and conditions in which bowel rhythm and function are upset. They have a traditional use in treating premature ejaculation in men, and the sedative effect may be complemented by a hormonal influence brought about by hops.

Dosage and preparations
Tincture – 1:5, 60%, 1–2 ml.
Infusion – 0.5–1 g per cup.
Should be fairly fresh for digestive properties; can be made into hops pillows when older, as volatile sedative substances accumulate.

Cautions and contraindications
Medicinal amounts should be used only with a doctor's supervision. Do not use in cases of depression. Hops can cause rashes, diarrhea, and stomachache in some people.

Hydrastis canadensis GOLDENSEAL

A small plant native to North America, goldenseal likes damp, shaded woodlands and is extremely difficult to cultivate. The root is harvested after five years and is usually used powdered, but may then be mixed with barberry bark, a relative. Expense and scarcity make it advisable to use alternatives until it can be grown and harvested more successfully. Goldenseal contains alkaloids, which seem responsible for most of its actions.

Actions Goldenseal is a powerful antiseptic and is astringent and healing to the gut wall and other mucous membranes. Often included in prescriptions for the lungs, reproductive tract, and kidneys, goldenseal is also a bitter digestive stimulant, a liver tonic, and cholagogue.

Uses Internally, goldenseal is excellent for catarrhal complaints of all kinds, but as it is cooling in nature, it should be combined with warming remedies such as ginger and cinnamon. It is one of the most widely used herbs for inflammation of the digestive tract. It is antibacterial and antifungal, and an infusion can bring topical relief to irritated eyes, lips, mouth, and throat.

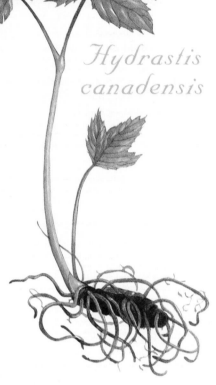

Hydrastis canadensis

Dosage and preparations
Tincture – 1:10, 60%, 0.5–2 ml.
Infusion – up to 1 g.

Cautions and contraindications
Pregnant women and people at risk for heart disease, diabetes, glaucoma, or stroke should not use goldenseal. Large doses can cause vomiting and breathing difficulty.

Hyssopus officinalis HYSSOP

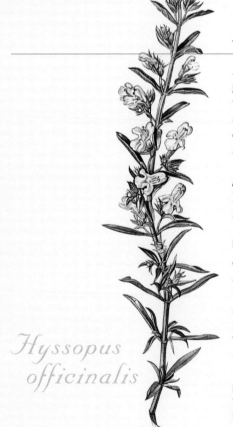

Hyssopus officinalis

An upright herb with attractive blue or pink flowers, hyssop is often grown in gardens. Its name means "holy herb," and Jewish priests used it to cleanse temples and other sacred sites in Jerusalem more than 2,500 years ago. The ancient Greeks made a syrup using hyssop, water, and honey to relieve chest congestion. Hyssop is rich in volatile oil and also contains bitter substances and tannins. It has a strongly aromatic odor and taste.

Actions Hyssop is sedative, diaphoretic, relaxing, and expectorant. Research has demonstrated that hyssop has an action that soothes mucous membranes and is an expectorant as well.

Uses Hippocrates recommended hyssop for chest complaints, and it is still considered useful for colds, chest infections, bronchial congestion, and asthma. For tight, dry, wheezy coughs it is even more effective when combined with marsh mallow or coltsfoot. It is an excellent herb for children, specifically for overexcitability and asthma with a nervous component. A hyssop infusion is relaxing and makes a pleasant tea for nervous exhaustion. The essential oil, applied diluted, has an antiviral effect and can help combat the herpes simplex virus.

Dosage and preparations
Tincture – 1:5, 45%, 1–2 ml.
Infusions – 1–2 g.

Cautions and contraindications
Do not use in large doses.

Hypericum perforatum ST. JOHN'S WORT

St. John's wort is a shrub that is native to Europe, western and northern Asia, and northern Africa, but now grows widely across North America. It is distinguishable from many of its close relatives by its small oval leaves, which are punctured by translucent dots. The leaves and flowers are harvested in summer. Surprisingly, the yellow flowers yield a deep red juice, and the herb also contains flavonoid glycosides and tannins.

Actions In Germany a standardized extract of St. John's wort has been extensively used and researched as an herbal antidepressant, and it is now among the biggest-selling medicines in that country. In clinical trials it has proved as effective for mild to moderate depression as major synthetic drugs, but without their side effects. In the Middle Ages, St. John's wort was used as a major wound healer, particularly for deep sword wounds. It promotes tissue regeneration and is antibacterial, astringent, and antispasmodic. Hypericin, the red pigment found particularly in the oil, is thought to have an antiviral action and is under investigation as a treatment for HIV infection.

Uses The main use of St. John's wort has been in the treatment of moderate depression, and it has been found so effective that the mood-lifting effects become apparent after only two weeks of treatment. Herbalists prescribe St. John's wort more as a nervous system restorative than as simply an antidepressant, however, and use it for many conditions associated with nervous stress—insomnia, anxiety, bed-wetting, and colic, for example. St. John's wort can be of great benefit in treating menopausal complaints, such as mood swings, irritability, and low energy. The herb's antispasmodic and relaxing effects make it useful for digestive complaints marked by nervous tension. Externally, the oil's healing and mild analgesic properties help to ease the pain caused by arthritis, neuralgia (nerve irritation), and shingles, and help to soothe burns, wounds, and hemorrhoids.

Dosage and preparations
Tincture – 1:5, 45%, 2–4 ml.
Infusion – 2–5 g per cup.
To make the infused oil, collect the flowers in June or July and pack them into a jar containing sunflower oil. Leave on a sunny windowsill for at least two weeks, and then press out and filter the oil, which will have turned a deep red color because of the hypericin in it.

Cautions and contraindications
St. John's wort can trigger a temporary photosensitive skin rash; exposure to sunlight should be limited while using it. People with high blood pressure, pregnant and nursing women, and anyone taking MAO inhibitors should avoid the herb. It is advisable to use St. John's wort only under medical supervision.

Hypericum perforatum

Inula helenium ELECAMPANE

A large herb, growing up to 3 m (10 ft), elecampane is native to central Europe and Asia but now grows in North America. The rhizomes of two- or three-year-old plants are usually collected in spring or autumn. They contain both a volatile oil and a bitter principle and are dried at a low temperature because the volatile oil is easily lost. Elecampane, which has a distinctive, aromatic flavor, was a common ingredient in many digestive liqueurs and old-fashioned cough candies.

Actions Elecampane is expectorant and antitussive and supports digestive and eliminatory functions. Certain components of the essential oil stimulate the tissues of the digestive tract, which in turn stimulate a reflex in the respiratory and urinary systems. This stimulation and reflex help to liquefy secretions, thus aiding elimination of waste.

Uses Excellent for relieving chronic coughs, particularly in the elderly, elecampane is also useful for relieving digestive problems and was traditionally used as an anthelmintic. It is also applied externally for scabies, herpes, and other skin infections and infestation.

Dosage and preparations
Best prepared fresh.
Tincture – 1:5, 45%, 2–4 ml.
Infusion/cold decoction – 1–3 g per cup.

Cautions and contraindications
Pregnant and nursing women, diabetics, and children under age two should avoid using the herb. Elecampane can cause allergic reactions of the skin. Large doses can cause vomiting, diarrhea, dizziness, and spasms.

Inula helenium

Juniperus communis JUNIPER

An evergreen shrub often seen on exposed wasteland slanting away from the prevailing wind, juniper is widely distributed throughout the Northern Hemisphere and is common in North America. The berries are harvested from September to October and are used as a flavoring for gin as well as for their medicinal properties.

Actions Juniper is diuretic, antiseptic—especially for the urinary tract—assists elimination of uric acid and is a relaxing digestive tonic. External applications stimulate the circulation.

Uses Juniper is a powerful urinary antiseptic for cystitis and a stimulating cleanser for indigestion, rheumatism, tendon problems, gout, and neuralgia. Externally, the diluted essential oil is an excellent rub or bath for tight muscles and rheumatic pain.

Dosage and preparations
Tincture – 1:5, 45%, 1–2 ml.
A few berries can be eaten raw or infused, fresh or dried.
For external use, the essential oil may be mixed up to 5% in a base oil. Infused oil can be made by macerating 100 g of crushed berries in 1 liter of oil for 15 days in sunlight.

Cautions and contraindications
Do not use during pregnancy or if suffering from kidney disease. Do not take juniper for more than six weeks in a row. The oil may cause gastric irritation, diarrhea, and kidney damage.

Juniperus communis

Laurus nobilis BAY

Bay, also known as laurel and bay laurel, is a native of Mediterranean countries, where it grows up to 18 m (60 ft). The species cultivated in North America is much smaller and is often grown in a pot. The leaves are popular as a flavoring for sauces and the oil is sometimes used in perfumery.

Actions The essential oil extracted from bay leaves has antiseptic, antifungal, and rubifacient properties.

Uses The infused oil makes an excellent rub for general aches and pains, rheumatic complaints, sprains, and bruises. Either a tincture or some freshly crushed leaves may help heal minor scrapes and cuts.

Dosage and preparations
One or two leaves used in stews and soups to strengthen digestion. Tincture – 1:5, 45%, applied topically.

Cautions and contraindications
Do not use bay during pregnancy. If you are picking your own bay leaves be sure you have the correct species; mountain laurel (*Kalmia latifolia*), which looks very similar, is poisonous. Contact dermatitis may result from using bay externally. It should be taken internally in moderation.

Laurus nobilis

Lavandula officinalis LAVENDER

Native to southern Europe, lavender is cultivated throughout North America as a border or hedging plant in gardens for its flowers, its attraction for bees, and its pleasing smell. The flowers contain tannins and a gentle essential oil.

Actions A sedative and antidepressant, lavender is also carminative, mildly spasmolytic, and cholagogue. The volatile oil is anti-infective, rubefacient, antirheumatic, and healing, especially for burns. It is also sedative when applied to the skin and very effective in a bath.

Uses The infusion or tincture is useful for excitability, headaches, nervous palpitations, and insomnia. It is also very helpful for colic and for digestive problems of a nervous origin. The volatile oil, as long as it is of good quality, is both healing and disinfecting, making it extremely useful for burns, fungal skin disorders, and other skin infections. You can also use it externally or in an oil vaporizer for respiratory infections and for ear infections in children if the drum is not perforated.

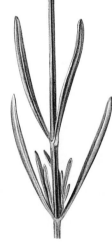

Lavandula officinalis

Dosage and preparations
Tincture – 1:5, 45%, up to 2 ml.
Infusions can be used topically (10 g) or internally (1–2 g).
Infused oil – make in a sealed, transparent container and leave in sunlight for a week.
Essential oil – dilute to 10–25%. May be applied undiluted to burns.

Cautions and contraindications
Lavender can be poisonous when taken internally. Pregnant women should never ingest it, and others should be medically supervised.

Leonurus cardiaca MOTHERWORT

This dark green, bushy plant, with toothed leaves and whorls (rings) of pale pink flowers, is found in hedgerows across temperate regions. Motherwort has a traditional use in midwifery to increase contractions and help expel the placenta. It contains alkaloids and bitter glycosides.

Actions Motherwort is a gentle uterine stimulant and relaxant. Modern research has indicated possible effects in calming the heart and lowering blood pressure.

Uses Motherwort has three spheres of influence: nervous, circulatory, and uterine. It is used for delayed, painful, or irregular menstruation, especially associated with nervous tension, and as a regulator during menopause. Motherwort is traditionally used to treat palpitations and is helpful for the nervous or hormonal problems that may underlie this complaint in women. It is best, however, to seek professional help, as palpitations occasionally indicate heart problems for which mother-wort may not be adequate treatment.

Leonurus cardiaca

Dosage and preparations
Tincture – 1:5, 25%, 2–5 ml.
Infusion – 2–4 g per cup.

Cautions and contraindications
Avoid use during pregnancy or lactation. Do not use in conjunction with other heart medications. Some people may experience an allergic reaction to motherwort.

Levisticum officinale LOVAGE

Levisticum officinale

Garden lovage is a member of the carrot family and has a sweet, aromatic taste, somewhere between those of celery and angelica. It is one of the old English herbs much used in cooking and is excellent in tomato soup. The root, and to a lesser extent the leaves and seeds, is used medicinally and contains a volatile oil. Lovage also has a bitter principle and contains benzoic acid, resins, and sitosterols, which are similar to some of the steroidal hormones found naturally in the body.

Actions Like angelica (see page 92), lovage is a warming digestive tonic and an effective carminative. It is diaphoretic, antimicrobial, and expectorant, a gentle diuretic, and like many anti-spasmodic plants, is also an emmenagogue.

Uses Lovage is helpful for indigestion and flatulence, especially in conjunction with poor appetite. A hot lovage infusion is good for colds and as an expectorant for bronchial infections. Because of its antimicrobial action, lovage is a useful gargle and mouthwash for treating sore throats and mouth ulcers. It is also diuretic and is used to treat urinary infections.

Dosage and preparations
Tincture – 1:5, 45%, 0.5–2 ml.
Infusion – 1 g per cup, in water or milk, and five times that strength as a mouthwash or gargle.

Cautions and contraindications
Lovage should be avoided by pregnant women and people with kidney disease. It may cause sensitivity to sunlight.

Mahonia aquifolium OREGON GRAPE

Oregon, or mountain, grape is a shrub with holly-shaped leaves that is native to the Pacific Northwest. Elsewhere it is a popular garden plant.

Actions Oregon grape can be used as a tissue cleanser, an alterative, and a digestive stimulant. Recent research has shown that it can inhibit some types of lipid breakdown in the body, which contribute to the inflammation of psoriasis. It may also be an important antifungal agent for the gut, due to the action of the alkaloid berberine.

Uses The dried roots and rhizomes are used for chronic skin, joint, and other inflammatory problems and can be used topically for psoriasis. The herb has long had a reputation as one of the main alterative or cleansing herbs and is a staple in prescriptions for eczema and psoriasis. Recently Oregon grape has been used to treat fungal overgrowth in the gut and other conditions associated with this problem. Oregon grape's bitter and cholagogue effects are useful for poor appetite, sluggish digestion, and poor liver function.

Mahonia aquifolium

Dosage and preparations
Tincture – 1:5, 25%, 2–4 ml.
Decoction – 1–2 g per cup, simmered for 20 minutes.

Cautions and contraindications
Do not take during pregnancy.

Malus spp. APPLE

Apple trees grow throughout Europe and North America. The fruits are a very healthy food, as folk wisdom has always held, and eating two apples a day over several weeks has been shown to reduce levels of cholesterol. The practice also appears to shift the profile of lipids in the blood away from the dangerous low-density types (LDLs) to the safer high-density ones (HDLs). This is particularly true for many people with a genetic tendency to high cholesterol and, for an unknown reason, for women.

Malus spp.

Dosage and preparations
To make the most of all the beneficial effects of apples, they are best eaten fresh and unpeeled. Apples should be washed carefully before eating.

Cautions and contraindications
Unripe or unpeeled apples can exacerbate chronic diarrhea in children and irritable bowel syndrome in some adults.

Actions Apples are good for people with diabetes because they help to stabilize blood sugar, providing sustained release of sugars in the blood without the sudden rise (followed by an insulin surge and low blood sugar) caused by eating sugary foods. The polyphenols, which are concentrated in and under the peel, are antiviral and may help reduce the risk of some cancers.

Uses Apples are also helpful in regulating bowel movements and are traditionally believed to aid the digestion of fatty foods; hence the custom of serving applesauce with roast pork.

Melissa officinalis LEMON BALM

A familiar lemon-scented garden herb, lemon balm is a favorite with bees (*melissa* comes from the Greek word for bee). It is harvested just before flowering, in the early afternoon, when the volatile oil content peaks. As well as volatile oil, lemon balm contains tannins and a bitter principle.

Actions Lemon balm is a relaxant with antispasmodic, carminative, and mildly diaphoretic properties. It has been used "to make the heart merry" since ancient times. Clinical trials have demonstrated lemon balm's ability to calm nervous tension, probably thanks to absorption of the volatile oil by emotional centers in the midbrain. Infusions applied topically have shortened the healing time of herpes lesions. The diluted essential oil helps relieve the pain of shingles, heal wounds, and soothe insect bites.

Uses This is an excellent herb for restlessness, agitation, and irritability, especially associated with neuralgia, headaches, palpitations, or gastric upset. Take plentifully after a meal as a relaxing digestive and before bed to prevent insomnia and nightmares.

Dosage and preparations
Tincture – 1:5, 45%, 2–5 ml.
Infusion – 2–4 g or 2 fresh leaves per cup.
For shingles or neuralgia, use 5% essential oil in a cream or base oil.

Cautions and contraindications
Lemon balm is generally a safe herb and well suited to children. People with thyroid problems should consult a doctor before using lemon balm.

Melissa officinalis

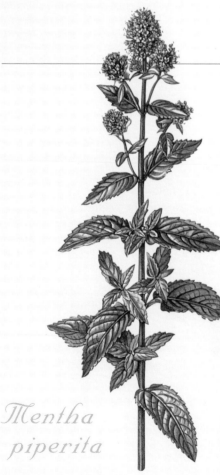

Mentha piperita PEPPERMINT

Peppermint, but one of about 25 mint species and hundreds of varieties and hybrids, all of which share common characteristics, is a hybrid of water mint (*M. aquatica*) and spearmint (*M. spicata*); this last has been used medicinally since at least the time of the ancient Egyptians. Peppermint and spearmint are the two most popular mints in North America. The leaves are harvested just before the plant flowers and contain a volatile oil that is rich in menthol, plus flavonoids, phenolic acids, tanninlike substances, and a bitter principle.

Actions Peppermint is an aromatic digestive stimulant; the flavonoids are mildly antispasmodic and the oil is powerfully antispasmodic, carminative, and cholagogue. Peppermint oil is strongly antibacterial, antiprotozoal, and drying when inhaled. Topically, it is cooling and anesthetic when very dilute, but in higher concentration causes heat and redness.

Uses Peppermint is a useful remedy for colic, diarrhea, sluggish digestion, flatulence, and nausea. A hot infusion helps to relieve the sore throat of a cold, and the essential oil can be inhaled for congested catarrh of the sinuses and bronchial tubes. At concentrations of 0.5–1 percent, the oil soothes painful and itchy eczema, neuralgia, shingles, psoriasis, and rheumatic pain. Peppermint also aids the healing of stomach ulcers.

Mentha piperita

Dosage and preparations
Tincture – 1:5, 45%, 10–20 drops.
Infusion – 2–4 g per cup, between and after meals.

Cautions and contraindications
Use as an inhalant for short periods only. Do not give the tea to babies. Avoid medicinal use if you have gallbladder problems or liver damage. Do not use the essential oil during pregnancy.

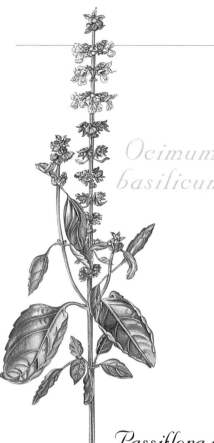

Ocimum basilicum BASIL

Basil is now used mainly for cooking, but for many centuries it was an important medicinal plant across the world. It is a nonhardy annual that grows in warm climates and likes a sunny location. The medicinal properties lie in the leaves, which contain a volatile oil and vitamins A and C.

Actions Basil is a nervous restorative and antidepressant. It is mildly sedative and is a reputed stimulant for the adrenal system, which regulates hormone levels. The volatile oil is strongly anti-infective and has a decongestant and antispasmodic action. It can also be used as a carminative and a galactagogue and is an aromatic, digestive stimulant with some vermicidal activity.

Uses Inhalations of the essential oil are useful for clearing and disinfecting the sinuses and air passages during head colds and chest infections. Basil is a useful herb to take when depressed or in low spirits, and it combines well with lemon balm. It is also used to improve sluggish digestion and relieve gas. Its antiseptic quality makes it suitable to put on cuts and insect bites.

Dosage and preparations
Basil is more effective in the form of a tincture (1:5, 45%, 1–3 ml) than as an infusion. The fresh leaves (far superior to the dried) can be eaten regularly in salads as a nerve tonic – 1–3 leaves per day will suffice.

Cautions and contraindications
Pregnant and nursing women should avoid medicinal doses of basil. (Culinary amounts should not interfere with pregnancy.) Do not give basil to infants or toddlers.

Passiflora incarnata PASSIONFLOWER

This woody and exotic climbing vine is a native of the southeastern United States and Central and South America. Jesuit priests saw elements of the crucifixion in the flowers and so gave it the name passionflower. Its aerial parts are collected and dried for medicinal use after the edible passion fruits have been harvested. The herb contains useful alkaloids and flavonoids.

Actions Passionflower has a mild sedative effect, thought to derive from its flavonoids, which have some of the same pharmacological effects as the widely used prescription sedative diazepam, but without the side effects. Its anodyne and antispasmodic properties are thought to be derived from other constituents.

Uses This is one of the most popular herbs for the self-treatment of neuralgia, restlessness, irritability, excitability, and insomnia. Although passionflower is not always strong enough to use by itself for encouraging sleep, it is useful in supporting the actions of other sedatives, such as hops and valerian. Although based only on animal studies, the influential and ongoing German Commission E report on herbal remedies recommends passionflower for nervous agitation. Passionflower has also been found to give partial relief from the pain of shingles and hemorrhoids.

Dosage and preparations
Tincture – 1:5, 25%, 2–4 ml.
Infusion – 1 g per cup, steeped for 5 minutes.

Cautions and contraindications.
Pregnant women should not use passionflower.

Passiflora incarnata

Petroselinum crispum PARSLEY

Indigenous to the eastern Mediterranean, parsley has been widely cultivated since the time of the ancient Greeks; it flourishes in a sunny location and rich, limy soil. Two-year-old roots and leaves are used medicinally and contain volatile oil, flavonoids, vitamins A and C, and iron, calcium, phosphorus, and manganese.

Actions Parsley is diuretic, nutritive, carminative, and antispasmodic. It is also a stomachic and general stimulant to the digestive organs, as well as being a useful breath freshener.

Uses Parsley is very useful for relieving water retention, and its digestive stimulating properties make it a good general cleanser for congested conditions. It is indicated in anemia and nutritional deficiency because of its mineral content and is excellent for poor appetite and digestion and for flatulence and colic. A sprig of parsley is also very effective for reducing garlic breath.

Dosage and preparations
Tincture – 1:5, 45%, 2–5 ml.
Infusion – 2 g per cup, covered and steeped for 5 minutes.
Decoction of root – 3–4 g per cup, covered and simmered for 20 minutes. For nutritional deficiency, add sprigs of fresh parsley to salads.

Cautions and contraindications
Avoid taking medicinal amounts of parsley during pregnancy and if you are suffering from any form of kidney disease. Parsley may cause an allergic reaction such as sensitivity to light.

Petroselinum crispum

Phytolacca americana POKEROOT

Pokeroot—also known by nearly two dozen other common names, including poke, pokeweed, pokeberry, and inkberry—is a strikingly tall perennial that produces drooping clusters of red berries. It is indigenous to eastern North America but has become naturalized in Europe, and prefers damp, shady conditions. The dried root contains saponins, alkaloids, and resins.

Actions Poke has a long-standing reputation as a powerful lymphatic alterative and stimulant. It also stimulates elimination and possibly has an action that stimulates white blood cell activity.

Uses This was an important herb for shamanistic practitioners of North America in the 19th century, who used it for a wide range of infectious and congestive disorders, including relief of rheumatic pain and swollen lymph nodes and other conditions affecting lymphatic and glandular tissues, such as mumps, tonsillitis, and swollen adenoids. It was also used to treat chronic skin conditions, such as acne, and as a poultice for mastitis. Because all parts of the plant are toxic, however, it is no longer recommended for use.

Dosage and preparations
Tincture – 1:5, 25%, 5–10 drops.
Decoction – 0.5 g per day, simmered in a cup of water for 20 minutes.

Cautions and contraindications
Ingestion of the plant can cause severe stomach cramps, diarrhea, difficulty breathing, vomiting, spasms, severe convulsions, and death.

Phytolacca americana

116

Plantago spp. PLANTAIN (PSYLLIUM)

There are some 250 species of plantain, a low to medium-size hardy perennial with single stems that each bear a spike of tiny gray-brown flowers. It is widely distributed around the Northern Hemisphere, especially in grasslands and by fresh water, and is very difficult to eradicate from lawns. Plantain was much used by the Anglo-Saxons as a laxative and for bites and wounds. The leaves and seeds contain mucilage, tannins, and minerals such as zinc, silica, and potassium.

Actions Plantain is laxative, mildly astringent, and healing, with styptic and demulcent properties. Ribwort plantain is widely used by herbalists as an anticatarrhal tonic and a relaxing expectorant.

Uses Plantain is an excellent restorative for all forms of respiratory congestion—nasal catarrh, bronchitis, sinusitis, and middle ear infections. Plantain's demulcent quality makes it useful for painful urination. Topically, it calms the irritation and itching of insect bites, stings, and skin irritations, and acts as a disinfectant and styptic for wounds. The seeds of *P. psyllium* are an effective laxative.

Dosage and preparations
Tincture – 1:5, 25%, 2–5 ml.
Infusion – 2–3 g per cup, infused for 5 minutes. Both the fresh juice and tincture are styptic but this property is inactivated by heating.

Cautions and contraindications
The seeds should not be used in cases of intestinal obstruction and should not be given to children under age two. Avoid excessive use during pregnancy.

Rheum palmatum CHINESE RHUBARB

Chinese rhubarb is indigenous to the hilly areas of central and eastern Asia. Greek physicians who obtained rhubarb from caravans plying trade routes to the Orient used it to promote menstruation, heal burns and sores, and clear the bowels. Rhubarb root contains anthraquinones (which are strongly laxative), tannins, and bitters.

Actions In very small doses rhubarb is an astringent digestive tonic, stimulating liver and gallbladder function; in larger doses it is purgative.

Uses Chinese rhubarb can be taken for sluggish digestion and diarrhea in small doses and for occasional constipation in larger amounts. It has been used to treat bacterial dysentery. (It may stimulate the body's natural means of ridding itself of the bacteria, or its tannins, which are antibacterial, may be the effective component.) English rhubarb *(Rheum officinale)* is used as a tonic for estrogen deficiency, particularly for women during the menopause.

Dosage and preparations
Tincture – 1:5, 25%, 0.5–4 ml.
Powder – 0.1–1 g daily.

Cautions and contraindications
Do not take rhubarb during pregnancy or while nursing or if you are suffering from gout or arthritis. Also refrain from using it if bowel obstruction is suspected or abdominal pain is present. The leaves are poisonous.

Rosa spp. ROSE

Roses were originally native to the eastern Mediterranean, where they were widely used in decorative, ceremonial, and symbolic functions more than 2,500 years ago. They are now cultivated worldwide for their beauty, as well as for the sweet, intensely fragrant oil extracted from the petals, which contain nerol, geraniol, and other constituents. Rose hips, which are gathered mainly from the dog rose (*Rosa canina*) are rich in vitamin C. Rose hips also contain tannins, flavonoids, and mucilage.

Actions The petals of roses have antispasmodic, sedative, and astringent properties. They are a topical antiseptic and a gentle laxative. They can also help to regulate the menstrual cycle and are anti-inflammatory. Rosewater is a gentle skin cleanser and the basis of a skin-protective cream. Rose hip tea can be used to relieve and treat scurvy and is mildly astringent and diuretic.

Uses Rose hip tea is an old folk remedy for colds and mild diarrhea. Rose petals make a pleasant, soothing, and anti-inflammatory infusion, which is helpful for digestive debility, respiratory and gastrointestinal infestations, and mild inflammations of the mouth and pharynx. Some herbalists believe it can also alleviate mild depression and anxiety. The oil, which is very expensive and worth using only if unadulterated, also reduces inflammation and fights fungal infection.

Rosa spp.

Dosage and preparations
Infusion – 1 g petals per cup. Fresh petals give best results.

Cautions and contraindications
The essential oil should not be used during pregnancy.

Rosmarinus officinalis ROSEMARY

This aromatic kitchen herb is indigenous to maritime regions of southern Europe and thrives on sandy soil in open sunlight. It has historical associations with remembrance and fidelity. Sprigs of rosemary were traditionally exchanged in a gesture of friendship, thrown into graves in commemoration, and worn in the hair to sharpen recollection. In addition to its volatile oil, rosemary contains flavonoids, a bitter principle, and a resin.

Actions Rosemary is a stimulating tonic that increases blood flow to the peripheries of the body and the brain, at the same time strengthening capillary walls. It is warming and drying and helps to stimulate the circulation while being antispasmodic. Externally, it has an anodyne effect on muscle and joint rheumatism. Internally, it is an aromatic digestive stimulant, increasing the flow of bile. Rosemary is strongly antibacterial and antifungal.

Uses Rosemary is good for mild depression associated with nervous tension, particularly when combined with lavender and taken internally or in a bath. It is also useful for migraines and tension headaches that are relieved by heat, and for indigestion, poor appetite, and flatulence. Used as a hair rinse, the infusion diminishes dandruff and hair loss.

Rosmarinus officinalis

Dosage and preparations
Tincture – 1:5, 45%, 1–3 ml.
Infusion – 2–4 g of dried herb, used mainly in combination with other herbs.

Cautions and contraindications
Avoid medicinal quantities during pregnancy. Do not use undiluted rosemary oil.

Rubus idaeus RASPBERRY

Raspberry grows wild in much of Europe and North America. It likes a rich, loamy soil and can be cultivated by planting suckers 60–90 cm (2–3 ft) apart, with about 1.5 m (4–5 ft) spaces between rows. The leaves contain tannins and an alkaloid, and the fruit is rich in vitamin C and minerals.

Actions Astringent and toning to the uterine and pelvic muscles.

Uses Raspberry leaf tea is famous for increasing the strength of contractions during childbirth and making delivery easier; for this purpose the tea should be taken 2 or 3 times daily in the last 3 months of pregnancy. Traditionally, it was combined with motherwort (see page 112) for threatened miscarriage. As an astringent remedy, the infusion is a useful treatment for diarrhea in children. Raspberry leaf tea can also be used as a gargle or mouthwash for mouth ulcers, oral thrush, and sore throats, or as a lotion for diaper rash, and it is a popular remedy for painful menstrual periods and premenstrual syndrome.

Rubus idaeus

Dosage and preparations
Tincture – 1:5, 25%, 5-10 ml.
Infusion – 5 to 8 g per cup.

Cautions and contraindications.
A pregnant woman should consult her doctor before taking the tea.

Salix alba WILLOW

Salix alba

The dried bark of this common tree is collected from young branches during the growth period. Willow bark is famous for containing aspirin-like substances—phenolic glycosides, including salicylates. It also contains flavonoids and tannins. Being very strong and supple, willow twigs have many domestic uses.

Actions Willow is anti-inflammatory, analgesic, antipyretic, antirheumatic, and astringent. Interestingly, some of willow's active constituents, while sharing the pain-relieving effects of aspirin (acetylsalicylic acid), have a more sustained action in the body and fewer side effects than aspirin.

Uses Willow bark helps to reduce high fevers and to relieve the pain of arthritis and headaches. Although these claims have not been proven clinically, the indications are strongly supported by the fact that the bark was used in a way similar to that of aspirin long before the invention of the drug.

Dosage and preparations
Tincture – 1:5, 25%, up to 8 ml.
Decoction – 3–5 g per cup.

Cautions and contraindications
Avoid willow if you are sensitive to aspirin, have peptic ulcers, gout, asthma, diabetes, hemophilia, or kidney or liver disease.

Sambucus nigra ELDER

The elder is a small tree or shrub that grows in woods and on wasteland. It has stiff, pithy stems and produces flat heads of small creamy flowers in June, which give out a characteristic sweet, perfumed smell, and black berries in late summer and early autumn. Elder has a great number of folklore associations. It is featured, for example, in Arthurian tales, while a biblical legend holds that Judas hanged himself on the elder tree. Elder has long been associated with witch-craft and religion, which may partly reflect the wide range of medicinal uses of many parts of the plant. It is widely available and has a distinctive look. Today only the flowers and berries are used medicinally, and the berries are used in jellies, pies, pancakes, and fritters.

Sambucus nigra

Actions The flowers and berries of the elder are diaphoretic and expectorant. Elderflowers are used in particular to relieve catarrh and to improve the tone of nasal mem-branes. According to Dr. Fritz Weiss, the much respected German herbalist, elderflowers raise the resistance to respiratory infections. Recent laboratory tests in Israel showed that elderberry extract inhibits various strains of the influenza virus and, if taken early on in an attack of influenza, can dramati-cally improve recovery times. Both the berries and the flowers encourage the fever response and stimulate sweating, which prevents very high temperatures and provides an important channel for detoxification. In addition, the flowers are diuretic, while the berries are mildly laxative. The inner bark has a history of use as a purgative, dating back to the time of Hippocrates. An ointment made from elder flowers was once used for chilblains and stimulating local circulation.

Uses Traditional winter cold remedies using elder include elderberry wine, which should be taken hot and mixed with cinnamon; elderberry syrup, made by simmering down 2.5 kg (5 lb) of elderberries with 500 g (1 lb) of sugar; and elderflowers combined in a hot infusion with peppermint and yarrow. Elder leaves make a useful ointment for bruises, sprains, and wounds. Elderberry infusion is also useful as a gargle and mouthwash for colds. The flowers make popular hay fever treatments for their anticatarrhal properties, and their diuretic effect can also help to reduce fluid congestion.

Dosage and preparations
Tincture – 1:5, 25%, 1–5 ml.
Infusion – 1–3 g flowers per cup, can be taken frequently for colds or flu.

Cautions and contraindications
The raw berries are toxic; so too are formulas containing the root, leaf, bark, or stems.

Salvia officinalis SAGE

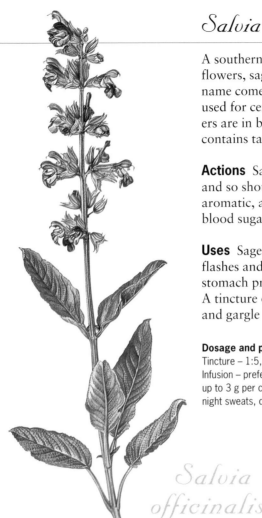

A southern European perennial with purple-green downy leaves and purple flowers, sage is widely grown as a potherb all across North America. The name comes from the Latin *salvere*, which means "to heal," and it has been used for centuries in this role. The aerial parts are harvested when the flowers are in bud; the small hairs (trichomes) contain a volatile oil. Sage also contains tannins, an estrogenic principle, a resin, and a bitter substance.

Actions Sage powerfully suppresses sweat secretion and milk production and so should be avoided by weaning mothers. It is astringent, antiseptic, aromatic, and stomachic. Sage has a long-standing reputation for reducing blood sugar and is traditionally seen as a restorative herb.

Uses Sage is a remedy for night sweats associated with fevers and hot flashes and other symptoms of menopause. It can also be very useful for stomach problems associated with poor digestion, and for poor circulation. A tincture or strong infusion of the fresh herb makes an ideal mouthwash and gargle for mouth ulcers, swollen gums, and sore throats.

Dosage and preparations
Tincture – 1:5, 45%, 10–30 drops. Infusion – preferably of the fresh herb, up to 3 g per cup. For hot flashes and night sweats, drink the infusion cold.

Cautions and contraindications
Avoid during pregnancy and breastfeeding. Sage oil must not be taken internally.

Salvia officinalis

Scrophularia nodosa FIGWORT

A tall, erect perennial with a sharply square stem—one country name for the plant is "carpenter's square"—figwort grows in moist areas of wasteland or cultivated ground throughout most of the Northern Hemisphere. The plant contains saponins, flavonoids, and resins.

Actions Figwort is a mild laxative, a lymphatic cleanser, and a diuretic. Its mild cardiac stimulatory action may be responsible for its reputation as a stimulant to the lymphatic system. Applied topically, figwort is mildly anodyne.

Uses Figwort is helpful for inflammatory skin conditions, such as eczema and psoriasis, especially when the condition is chronic and there is also discharge or swollen lymph nodes. The bruised leaves were traditionally used as a poultice and topically applied to relieve burns and swellings.

Dosage and preparations
Tincture – 1:5, 25%, 1–3 ml.
Infusion – up to 2 g per cup.

Cautions and contraindications
Figwort should be used internally only under strict medical supervision and should be avoided by people with heart conditions.

Scrophularia nodosa

Scutellaria spp. SKULLCAP

Skullcap has distinctive pairs of blue to pink flowers, serrated leaves, and seed capsules that look like helmets—hence its name. Another common name, mad-dog weed, derives from a claim made by an 18th-century doctor that it could cure rabies. The plant is a native of North America but is found widely across the world in temperate regions. Skullcap contains a bitter principle, flavonoid glycosides, tannins, and resins.

Actions The herb is relaxing, restorative, sedative, anticonvulsive, and antispasmodic. It also stimulates and strengthens digestion.

Uses The prime uses of skullcap are for nervous tension with exhaustion and debility, disturbed sleep, depression, fatigue, and headaches associated with overwork or worry. These reflect its reputation as a relaxing herb used for the nervous system. It has applications as a restorative and antispasmodic for a number of neurological and neuromotor conditions, including migraine and the effects of withdrawal from benzodiazepine tranquilizers taken for insomnia. Professionally, skullcap is prescribed to reduce the severity and frequency of epileptic attacks. In China skullcap has been found to inhibit the flu virus and is used to treat pneumonia.

Dosage and preparations
Tincture – 1:5, 25%, 2–6 ml.
Infusion – 1–2 g per cup, steeped for 5 minutes.

Cautions and contraindications
Large doses may cause giddiness, confusion, twitching, and seizures. Pregnant and nursing women and children under three should not take it. Medicinal use should be supervised by a physician.

Scutellaria spp.

Stellaria media CHICKWEED

A small, soft, trailing annual, chickweed has light green leaves and tiny white flowers and is generally found growing on wasteland, by roadsides, and as a weed on cultivated ground throughout temperate regions. Lightly boiled, chickweed resembles spinach; the fresh leaves can be used in salads. The plant contains anti-inflammatory saponins and mucilage.

Actions The herb is a mild expectorant with antipruriginous (anti-itching) and demulcent actions. It calms inflamed and itchy skin conditions.

Uses Chickweed has been used since time immemorial as a poultice and an ointment for inflamed skin conditions, especially when accompanied by itching, such as eczema, boils, abscesses, and insect bites. It is also a gentle expectorant for productive coughs.

Dosage and preparations
Best used fresh.
Tincture – 1:5, 25%, 3–5 ml.
Infusion – 2–4 g per cup.
For external use, an infused oil can be made or a strong infusion used as a lotion or combined with a cream.

Cautions and contraindications
None are known.

Stellaria media

Stachys officinalis BETONY

Betony is an upright herb with deep reddish purple flowers. According to Gerard's herbal: "Betony loves shadowie woods, hedge-rowes, and copses, the borders of pastures, and such like places." The aerial parts are harvested in July when the herb comes into flower. Betony contains tannins, a bitter principle, and alkaloids similar to those in yarrow and vervain.

Actions Betony is mildly diaphoretic and a circulatory stimulant for the head area. It is a general relaxant and restorative to the nervous system and a mild astringent, useful in cleaning and drying wounds. Betony is also a gentle bitter digestive and uterine stimulant.

Uses Betony has traditionally been used to treat a huge range of complaints. Augustus Caesar's physician listed no less than 47 diseases for which it was effective. The name is thought to derive from two Celtic words: *bew* ("head") and *ton* ("good"). Betony is an excellent herb for sinus congestion and headaches caused by problems in the sinuses and ears. It is also useful for headaches associated with nervous tension or debility.

Betony is a relaxing nervous restorative, especially suited to chronic, painful conditions, and is useful for relieving chronic insomnia. Hildegard von Bingen (see page 22) recommended betony for people prone to nightmares, and it had a long tradition of use in protecting people "against fearful visions," as Erasmus describes.

Betony can also be used as a cleansing herb, stimulating the liver and the circulation. In addition to its relaxant properties, it is excellent for sciatica and rheumatic complaints. The herb is also a useful tonic for sluggish digestion.

Betony and its relative woundwort (*Stachys palustris*) were once widely used to stanch the bleeding and promote the healing of open wounds. A compress of these herbs is helpful for minor cuts and bruises, bites, stings, and skin irritations. Both have also been used to relieve menstrual pain due to congestion associated with slow onset of menses.

Dosage and preparations
Tincture – 1:5, 25%, 2–4 ml.
Infusion – 1–3 g per cup.

Cautions and contraindications
Do not take during pregnancy. Large doses may cause diarrhea, and very large doses are emetic.

Stachys officinalis

Symphytum officinale COMFREY

A vigorous plant with broad, hairy leaves and drooping spikes of bell-shaped mauve or white flowers, comfrey grows on moist banks and in ditches throughout Europe and North America. The leaves and roots contain mucilage, tannins, and dangerous pyrrolizidine alkaloids.

Actions Comfrey is perhaps the most effective vulnerary herb of all, stimulating the cells that repair skin, connective tissue, and bone. It is demulcent and helps to soothe irritation and inflammation in the digestive tract. It is also an astringent and a relaxing expectorant.

Uses Comfrey is an excellent remedy for poorly healing skin, strains, sprains, and fractures (one of its common names, in fact, is knitbone). Both root and leaf have traditionally been used externally and internally for ulcers, gastritis, bronchitis, and irritable coughs, but because of the problems of toxicity from its alkaloids, which can cause liver damage, herbalists currently use the plant externally only.

Dosage and preparations
Tincture – (leaf) 1:5, 25%, 2–4 ml.
Infusion – (leaf) 2–3 g per cup.
Leaf and root can be used in ointments and poultices, infused oils, and creams.

Cautions and contraindications
Do not use comfrey internally nor apply it externally to large areas of broken skin. Products for internal use are not permitted to be sold in Canada, and Health Canada does not advise using skin care productsthat contain comfrey extracts. Pregnant and nursing women should avoid comfrey.

Symphytum officinale

Tanacetum parthenium FEVERFEW

Feverfew was brought to North America by English settlers and today grows throughout southern Canada and the United States. Since the 1970s it has become one of the most widely used herbal remedies in the Western world, but its usefulness in reducing fever and soothing arthritis pain and skin inflammations was already noted by the Greek physician Dioscorides in A.D. 78. The leaves and flowers are harvested during the summer months.

Actions Feverfew has anti-inflammatory and diaphoretic actions. Its efficacy in preventing and reducing the severity of migraine headaches has been well established. The active principles in feverfew, parthenolides, inhibit the release of serotonin, prostaglandins, and histamines into the bloodstream, all of which can inflame tissue, as well as trigger and worsen migraines.

Uses Feverfew has traditionally been used to treat fevers, calm the nerves, and relieve painful menstrual periods and rheumatic pains. A tincture or infusion of feverfew used topically will relieve the pain and swelling of insect bites and serve as an insect repellent.

Dosage and preparations
Tincture – 1:5, 25%, or of the fresh herb 1:2, 45%, 1–2 ml.
Infusion – 1 g per cup, steeped for 5 minutes.
Fresh leaf – two or three per day.
Tablets or capsules – one per day, containing no less than 0.2 percent parthenolides.

Cautions and contraindications
Feverfew should not be taken by pregnant women or children under age two. It can cause mouth ulcers, contact dermatitis, or stomach upsets in a small minority of people.

Tanacetum parthenium

Taraxacum officinale DANDELION

Dandelion is a highly adaptable plant thought to have originated in the foothills of central Asia, and is widely distributed throughout the Northern Hemisphere. The leaf and root are collected for medicinal purposes in spring. The root is also harvested in autumn when it is less bitter and higher in inulin, a kind of sugar. It is then roasted to make dandelion coffee.

The leaf and root contain vitamins A, C, and D and the B vitamins. The leaf is especially rich in potassium and vitamin A, and the root contains a large amount of starch. Both, but especially the root, contain a bitter latex—a milky kind of sap that becomes rubbery when dried. Indeed, a strain of dandelion was specially cultivated to augment the scarce and valuable supply of rubber needed to equip the Soviet army in the Second World War. Young leaves are refreshing in salads, and both the root and leaf have proved valuable foods in times of famine.

Actions Dandelion is a widely prescribed medicinal plant in Western herbalism, used to improve the removal of fluid waste and stimulate liver function. The liver is involved in most of the intricate metabolic pathways of the body, and herbalists see healthy liver activity as vital to the harmonious functioning of the digestive and eliminative processes. Dandelion leaf is a potent diuretic, yet also replaces the potassium that is lost from increased urine production, a common side effect of diuretics. The root is also a bitter digestive stimulant that promotes bile excretion and acts as a liver tonic and mild laxative.

Uses Dandelion relieves conditions in sluggish digestion and metabolism and works as a cleansing herb for gout, arthritis, and skin problems. A tonic made with the leaf has traditionally been given in spring to cleanse the system. The herb is used to treat bladder and kidney problems by reducing water retention. The latex of the stalk can help remove a wart; it must be dabbed on every day over several weeks, taking care not to touch the surrounding skin.

Taraxacum officinale

Dosage and preparations
Tincture – 1:5, 25%, 1–2 ml.
Infusions and decoctions – 3–10 g leaf or root per cup, 3–4 times daily.
Fresh juice of leaf and root – 3–5 ml.

Cautions and contraindications
Pregnant and nursing women and children under two should not drink dandelion tea. People with kidney, liver, bladder, stomach, and gallbladder problems are advised to consult a doctor before using dandelion. Internal use is contraindicated in bile-duct obstructions and gallstones.

Thymus vulgaris THYME

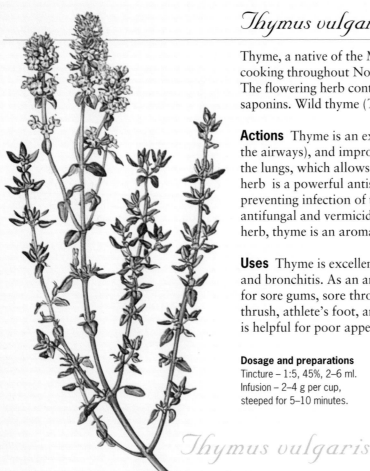

Thyme, a native of the Mediterranean, is grown in gardens and used in cooking throughout North America. It likes well-drained, lime-rich soil. The flowering herb contains volatile oil, tannins, bitters, flavonoids, and saponins. Wild thyme (*Thymus serpyllum*) has similar properties.

Actions Thyme is an expectorant, relaxes bronchial spasm (tightness of the airways), and improves fluid secretions. It is partly excreted through the lungs, which allows its healing properties to work directly there. The herb is a powerful antiseptic, making it useful for disinfecting cuts and preventing infection of the throat and lungs. Thyme essential oil is both antifungal and vermicidal (though nontoxic internally). As a digestive herb, thyme is an aromatic stimulant and carminative.

Uses Thyme is excellent for infectious or dry coughs, whooping cough, and bronchitis. As an antiseptic herb, it is a good mouthwash and gargle for sore gums, sore throats, and laryngitis. It is also a useful lotion for thrush, athlete's foot, and other fungal infections. As a digestive herb, it is helpful for poor appetite and flatulence.

Dosage and preparations
Tincture – 1:5, 45%, 2–6 ml.
Infusion – 2–4 g per cup, steeped for 5–10 minutes.

Cautions and contraindications
Thyme's essential oil should be well diluted for topical use and not used at all internally. Pregnant and nursing women and anyone with an overactive thyroid, colitis, or a heart problem should avoid medicinal amounts.

Thymus vulgaris

Tilia europea LINDEN

Linden trees, also known as lime or basswood, are large and leafy and commonly found throughout northern temperate zones. The flowers and bracts (leafy structures around the base of the flowers), present from May to July, are rich in flavonoids, saponins, mucilage, tannins, sugars, and a tiny amount of a substance similar to chemical tranquilizers.

Actions Linden flowers can be used as a sedative, a relaxant, an antispasmodic, and a vasodilator (an agent that widens and relaxes blood vessels). They are also diaphoretic and have diuretic properties.

Uses With their mild, pleasant taste, linden flowers (known as lime flowers in Europe) are popular herbal relaxants. They are useful in treating anxiety, migraine, and a range of circulatory problems, including palpitations and varicose veins. The saponins and flavonoids are thought to have a beneficial effect on the blood vessel walls in people with hardening of the arteries and high blood pressure. As a diaphoretic, linden is good for feverish colds and catarrh.

Tilia europea

Dosage and preparations
Tincture – 1:5, 25%, 1–2 ml.
Infusion – 2 tsp per cup, infused for no more than 5 minutes.

Cautions and contraindications
Excessive use of Linden may result in cardiac toxicity.

Trifolium pratense RED CLOVER

The flower heads of this familiar meadow plant are reddish purple, and the leaves consist of three oval leaflets. It is common throughout Europe and in central and eastern Asia. The flower heads contain flavonoids and a little volatile oil. Flavonoids in the leaves include several that act like the hormone estrogen, found naturally in the body.

Actions Though red clover is one of the most commonly used blood-cleansing herbs, its medicinal actions have not been thoroughly researched. It is prescribed by herbalists as a dermatological agent and alterative, a mild antispasmodic, and an expectorant.

Uses Externally, it is used to treat psoriasis, eczema, and other skin conditions. Used internally, it is a relaxing expectorant, helpful for relieving coughs, particularly whooping cough, and asthma. From the 1920s to the 1950s a red clover formula was used to treat cancer and was then banned.

Trifolium pratense

Dosage and preparations
Tincture – 1:5, 25%, in alcohol or glycerol, 2–5 ml.
Infusion – 2–4 g per cup.
An ointment for psoriasis can be made by boiling down a concentrated decoction until it reaches a thick, tarry consistency.

Cautions and contraindications
Pregnant and nursing women should avoid red clover. Large doses may interfere with anticoagulant and hormonal therapies.

Trigonella foenum-graecum FENUGREEK

Fenugreek is indigenous to the eastern Mediterranean but is cultivated extensively in other regions. Its seeds, used since antiquity as both food and medicine, appear in Chinese, Indian, Arabic, and Western herbal therapies. The seeds contain a volatile oil, mucilage, a bitter principle, steroidal saponins, and an alkaloid.

Actions Fenugreek seeds are a nutritive digestive tonic and, when moistened, are both demulcent and emollient. They have a long history of use as a galactagogue and also as a male hormonal tonic. Overall, fenugreek could be characterized as a strengthening herb that is also locally soothing.

Uses The seeds are useful for convalescent states, especially those involving poor digestion, and for painful bowel problems in which the mucilage acts to soothe and lubricate and to give the stool bulk and softness. Powdered and soaked overnight in water, fenugreek seeds can form a soothing, anti-inflammatory poultice for rheumatic pains, skin irritations, and abrasions. Fenugreek powder can be sprinkled directly on diaper rash to bring relief. An infusion or tincture increases milk production in nursing mothers and is used in China to treat impotence in men and menopausal problems in women. In the Middle East fenugreek is used to treat diabetes.

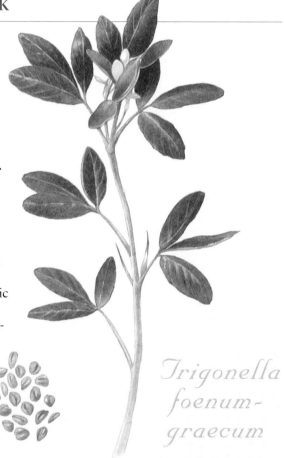

Trigonella foenum-graecum

Dosage and preparations
Tincture – 1:5, 45%, 2–4 ml.
Infusion – 2 g per cup, infused for 5 minutes.
Powder – as poultice.

Cautions and contraindications
Avoid during pregnancy.

Tussilago farfara COLTSFOOT

Coltsfoot grows in boggy ground or heavy clay. The single, hairy stem, covered in leaf scales, produces a bright yellow flower head in early spring. The leaves, to whose shape the name refers, reach full size in late spring. The leaves and flowers contain mucilage, and the leaves also contain tannins.

Actions Coltsfoot is a relaxing expectorant that is soothing to bronchial irritation and liquefying to bronchial secretions. The leaves are rich in zinc and potassium nitrate, burn well, and were the main ingredient of "cigarettes" the Romans used to treat asthma by inhaling the smoke through a reed. They are also vulnerary.

Uses A relaxing expectorant, useful for stubborn, tight coughs, for chronic chest problems, and asthma. Coltsfoot is an excellent cough suppressant, especially for smokers and elderly people. The leaves can be used in a poultice or ointment for cuts and poorly healing wounds.

Dosage and preparations
Tincture – 1:5, 25%, or fresh juice, 2–4 ml.
Infusion – 2–4 g leaves per cup.

Cautions and contraindications
Coltsfoot is now known to be dangerous in high concentrations, and several countries limit its content in herbal preparations. Internal use is discouraged, and external use should be limited to no more than six weeks a year. Pregnant and nursing women should avoid coltsfood entirely.

Tussilago farfara

Urtica dioica NETTLE

Stinging nettle is a large perennial that likes cultivated, nitrogen-rich soil and makes an excellent organic fertilizer. It is harvested in May and June, before flowering, while the stinging hairs on the leaves and stalk are rich in histamine and serotonin. The whole herb contains flavonoids, vitamins, and minerals, especially calcium and potassium salts and silicic acid.

Actions Nettles are excellent for regulating and optimizing bodily functions, and they are also a good cleansing and nutritive herb. Nettles cause increased elimination of sodium and urea, which is perhaps one reason why they have been found helpful for rheumatism and arthritis, because a buildup of these substances exacerbates these conditions. The fresh root is now widely prescribed for prostate hypertrophy (enlargement) and irritable bladders in older men.

Uses Nettles are helpful for skin problems and arthritis associated with poor circulation. They are also useful for allergic or irritable skin and respiratory problems, including asthma and urticaria (nettle rash). They have been used for centuries to promote milk production, both in humans and animals. A nettle infusion is a good spring cleansing tonic and a help in congestive conditions and water retention.

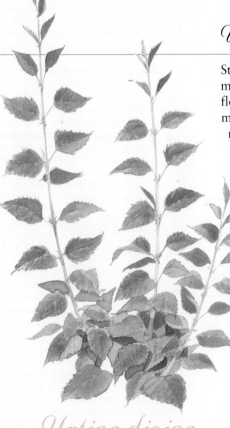

Urtica dioica

Dosage and preparations
Tincture – 1:5, 25%, 5 ml.
Infusion – 1–3 g per cup.
Fresh juice – 30 ml.

Cautions and contraindications
Pregnant women and children under two should not use nettle internally.

Vaccinium myrtillus BILBERRY

Bilberry grows in hilly areas of northern and central Europe (where it is sometimes called wild blueberry), Asia, and North America (where it is also known as Rocky Mountain blueberry). Bilberry is a small leathery-leaved shrub producing slightly acid-tasting berries that contain tannins, vitamin A, and a few minerals.

Actions Bilberry is astringent and antispasmodic with anti-inflammatory and mildly sedative properties. It is mildly antibacterial and the tannins probably account for its antidiarrheal action. Bilberry is also found in some remedies for improving poor night vision. The active constituents strengthen the capillaries and veins, improve peripheral circulation, and regulate the flow of blood.

Uses Only the berries are used. Bilberry is useful both as a treatment for diarrhea and as an herb to aid circulation, with particular application for eye problems, including cataracts, diabetic-induced glaucoma, poor night vision, and eyestrain. It is also used in association with circulatory or inflammatory conditions, such as allergic reactions, hypertension, poor circulation, and nerve and kidney problems resulting from fragile capillaries. Varicose veins are also relieved by bilberry.

Vaccinium myrtillus

Dosage and preparations
Tincture – 1:4, 25%, 5–10 ml.
Berries – fresh 2–4 g, dried 1 g.

Cautions and contraindications
Excessive doses of bilberry extracts are potentially toxic. They should be used only in moderation and for no longer than three weeks.

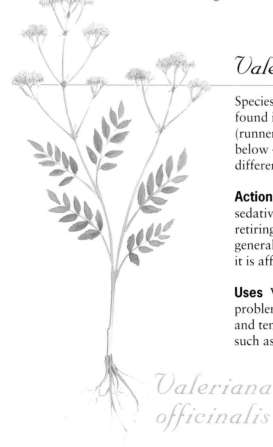

Valeriana officinalis VALERIAN

Species of valerian, a perennial that grows up to 1 m (3 ft) in height, are found in all temperate regions of the world. The rhizomes, roots, and stolons (runners) are harvested during the autumn and carefully dried at temperatures below 40°C. Valerian contains volatile oil and alkaloids. The combination of different constituents seems essential to its overall effects.

Actions The many studies of valerian's actions have established its mildly sedative, antispasmodic, and pain-relieving effects. Taken an hour before retiring, valerian shortens the time it takes to go to sleep and improves general sleep quality. The herb is also relaxing to the digestive system when it is affected by nervous tension.

Uses Valerian calms nervous tension and stress, nervous palpitations, skin problems that are exacerbated by anxiety or nervousness, nervous exhaustion, and tension headaches. It is also highly useful for nervous digestive problems, such as occasional constipation and irritable bowel syndrome.

Valeriana officinalis

Dosage and preparations
Tincture – 1:5, 45 %, 2–4 ml.
Infusion – 2–5 g, infused for 10 minutes.

Cautions and contraindications
Prolonged high doses of valerian can lead to irritability. A few people find that it gives them headaches. Pregnant and nursing women should avoid the herb. Children under age six should not be given valerian without medical supervision.

Verbascum thapsus MULLEIN

A tall biennial, common on dry roadsides and wasteland, mullein is densely covered with white woolly hairs. (The name *Verbascum* is derived from the Latin *barba*, meaning "beard.") The plant's long spikes of yellow flowers, which appear in the second year, used to be dipped in tar and used as a torch because the hairs were easily ignited. The leaves and flowers contain mucilage, saponins, flavonoids, and traces of volatile oil.

Actions Mullein is expectorant, demulcent, and a soothing diuretic.

Uses Excellent for coughs, especially tight, dry, and irritable types, mullein is specifically indicated for hoarseness, whooping cough, wheezy asthma, and bronchitis. The flowers are more strongly expectorant than the leaves, which are a soothing diuretic for irritation in the urinary tract. The infused oil, common in pharmacies as ear drops until recent times, is emollient and soothing and is used for earache and as a rub for inflamed joints. The bruised leaf is an old gardener's cure for hemorrhoids.

Dosage and preparations
Tincture – 1:5, 25%, 3–5 ml.
Infusion – 4–8 g of leaves or
1–4 g of flowers per cup.

Cautions and contraindications
Infusions should be carefully strained to filter out the fine hairs, which can irritate the throat. The plant's seeds are toxic.

*Verbascum
thapsus*

Verbena officinalis VERVAIN

A slender, erect perennial, bearing small lilac-colored flowers in long slender spikes, vervain grows by roadsides and in sunny pastures. (The species native to North America, *V. hastata*, has blue flowers.) The aerial parts are harvested just at flowering when they contain verbenalin, a bitter principle, tannins, flavonoids, and volatile oil.

Actions Mildly sedative, androgenic (increasing male hormones), emmenagogue, galactagogue, astringent, insecticidal, diaphoretic, vervain is a gentle and versatile favorite with many herbalists. Country names include simpler's joy and traveler's joy. In Germany it is known as ironwort because of its former use in treating wounds caused by iron weapons.

Uses Vervain is a calming restorative for debilitating conditions, particularly nervous exhaustion and depression. It is antiseptic to wounds and makes an excellent mouthwash for gum disease and a gargle for sore throat. It relieves poor menstrual flow and poor milk flow. In traditional Chinese medicine it is used as a blood detoxifier and for swollen throats.

Dosage and preparations
Tincture – 1:5, 25%, up to 5 ml.
Infusions – 2–4 g per cup; can
also be used as a lotion.

Cautions and contraindications
Pregnant women should avoid vervain because it is known to cause mild uterine contractions.

*Verbena
officinalis L.*

Viburnum opulus CRAMP BARK
Viburnum prunifolium BLACK HAW

Cramp bark, also known as highbush cranberry, snowball tree, and guelder rose, is a deciduous shrub native to North America and northern Europe. Similar in appearance to a small elder, the plant has flat-topped clusters of white flowers and large bright red berries similar to the cranberry so popular in sauces and breads. (The berries can be eaten, but only after cooking.) The bark contains a bitter resin and tannins. Black haw is also known by the common name cramp bark. A shrub indigenous to the United States, it is characterized by its short, pointed winter buds and sharply pointed leaves. Black haw berries are bluish black. The stem and root bark contain tannins and saponins.

Actions The two species are antispasmodic and are used to relieve menstrual cramping. Black haw also relieves the pain of headaches and arthritis because it contains salicin.

Uses Highbush cranberry is beneficial for conditions in which anxiety, muscular tension, and cramps are features. A strong infusion can be applied as a lotion for muscle cramps and spasms. Black haw is used more for menstrual problems, including threatened miscarriage, excessive menstrual bleeding, and pain.

Dosage and preparations
Tincture – 1:5, 25%, 3–8 ml.
Infusion – 1–3 g of dried powder, infused or simmered for 10 minutes.

Cautions and contraindications
Pregnant and nursing women and children under 16 should avoid black haw.

Viburnum prunifolium

Viburnum opulus

Vitex agnus-castus CHASTEBERRY

Chasteberry, also called agnus castus, is a Mediterranean shrub related to vervain. Its dried fruits have been used since antiquity to restrain sexual desire and nervous excitability. It contains a volatile oil, flavonoids, and a bitter principle.

Actions The berries of this plant shift the balance of hormones produced by the pituitary gland affecting the menstrual cycle. The overall effect of this shift is to increase the production of progesterone, leading to a reduction in premenstrual irritability, breast tenderness, and water retention.

Uses Chasteberry is one of the main herbal hormone tonics with a wide range of applications. It helps to regulate the menstrual cycle, especially frequent or heavy bleeding, and premenstrual symptoms such as breast tenderness and irritability. It promotes lactation in nursing mothers, helps reduce acne that is hormonally related, and encourages normal ovulation and menstruation, especially in women who have stopped taking birth-control pills. It can also reduce menopausal complaints, such as hot flashes.

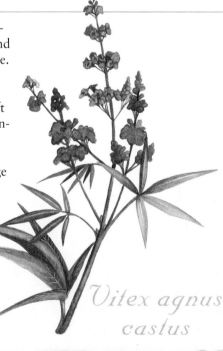

Vitex agnus castus

Dosage and preparations
Tincture – 1:5, 25%, 2–4 ml.
Powdered fruits – 0.3–1 g in the morning.

Cautions and contraindications
Use of chasteberry causes an itchy rash in some people.

Zea mays CORN SILK

Corn silk consists of the stigmas and styles (the silky strands emerging from the cob) of sweet corn, or maize. They contain insoluble sugars—mannitol, inositol, and sorbitol—a large amount of potassium, flavonoids, silica, and a small amount of volatile oil. Corn silk should be used fresh for best effect.

Actions Corn silk is a slightly demulcent soothing diuretic and a mild urinary antiseptic. Like dandelion leaf, it compensates for potassium lost through increased urine output because it has a high potassium content.

Uses An infusion taken several times a day soothes and calms the irritation of cystitis while helping to deal with the infection itself. It is not powerfully antiseptic and is best combined with antiseptic herbs like thyme and juniper. Its diuretic properties are helpful in treating edema, or water retention. Because of its soothing quality, it is also useful for relieving an irritable or nervous bladder, and as such is particularly recommended for helping to reduce bed-wetting in children.

Dosage and preparations
Tincture – 1:5, 25%, 2–4 ml.
Infusion – 2 g per cup.

Cautions and contraindications
None are known.

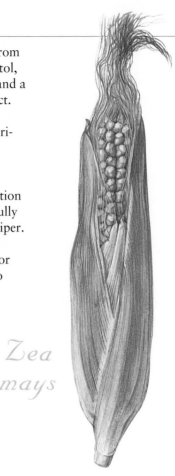

Zea mays

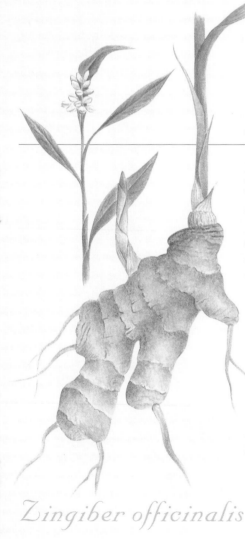

Zingiber officinale GINGER

Ginger is Asian in origin but widely cultivated in North America, the West Indies, India, and Africa. The root is used both fresh and dried and contains varying proportions of volatile constituents, depending on the area of origin and method of drying.

Actions Ginger is a strong circulatory stimulant with anticlotting, anti-inflammatory, and vasodilatory effects. It is a warming digestive stimulant and antispasmodic, an antiemetic, particularly when dried, and an antiseptic expectorant. The fresh root has a gentler, more peripheral action, while the dried root is a strong central stimulant with a more powerful digestive action. Ginger may help lower cholesterol, blood pressure, and the risk of blood clots, as well as fight intestinal infections and prevent ulcers.

Uses Ginger is a reliable travel sickness remedy and is helpful for poor digestion, especially accompanied by cold, and for colic, flatulence, and diarrhea. Ginger tea will help to sweat out a cold, is anticatarrhal, helpful for coughs, and eases menstrual cramps. It can also be of benefit for easing chronic inflammatory conditions such as arthritis (not during flare-ups, however), and improves circulation in cold hands and feet.

Dosage and preparations
Tincture – 1:5, 60%, 5–20 drops.
Candied ginger is helpful for nausea and travel sickness.

Cautions and contraindications
Ginger's use during pregnancy should be supervised by a doctor because it has an effect on the uterine muscles.

Zingiber officinalis

CHAPTER 6

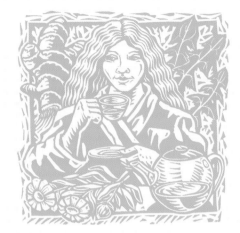

HEALING WITH HERBS

---

*Self-healing with herbs can be
effective, simple, and safe for many
minor conditions. From nausea to gout,
there is a selection of herbal remedies that
can be applied to offer speedy relief from
symptoms and hinder or prevent recurrence.
This chapter reveals a number of home
remedies that draw on the remarkable
secrets of herbal healing.*

Digestive system problems

Digestive disorders can range from uncomfortable heartburn to the more painful inflammation of colitis. Herbal preparations can help not only to relieve but also to prevent such problems.

When the body fails to digest food adequately or reacts to certain foods or events such as sea travel with diarrhea or nausea, the results can be highly discomforting. Some conventional treatments can be harsh on the system; herbal remedies often provide a gentler but equally effective alternative.

NAUSEA, VOMITING, AND MOTION SICKNESS

Nausea may be a sign of nervous tension or of something more serious, such as liver disease. It's not uncommon for it to occur in the early stages of pregnancy. In all these cases, the underlying cause of the condition should be diagnosed by a doctor and, whenever necessary, treated medically.

To deal with bouts of nausea when you are sure that the problem is benign and short-lived, such as motion sickness, you can use gingerroot. Fresh ginger is the traditional remedy for nausea and vomiting in both Ayurvedic and Tibetan medicine, and modern studies have confirmed its ancient uses. A fresh piece of the root chewed slowly is effective, or it may be drunk as a hot tea or eaten in the candied form. Ginger's advantage is that it does not cause drowsiness as some medications do.

Peppermint is another herb that has antiemetic properties, that is, counteracts nausea. Dried peppermint is widely available and is found in the form of teas, capsules, and tablets. Taken as tea, the herb is a quick antidote for a queasy stomach.

LOSS OF APPETITE AND WEAK DIGESTION

Although some people naturally have a weak digestion, an inexplicable loss of appetite may be a symptom of liver disease, an emotional problem such as depression, or the body's response to an acute illness. You should consult your doctor if you lose your appetite for more than three days.

HERBS AND THE DIGESTIVE SYSTEM

Many herbs act on the digestive system, either to soothe or stimulate, and herbal remedies can help to relieve many digestive disorders, from vomiting to gas.

Before you begin treatment, make sure you clearly understand your symptoms; some digestive disorders can indicate more serious underlying problems.

Gentian, mugwort, and centaury are recommended for loss of appetite.

Meadowsweet and marsh mallow are stomachic herbs that will relieve acid indigestion.

Licorice contains mucilage, which helps to relieve the pain of stomach ulcers.

Ginger and peppermint have antiemetic actions that help to relieve nausea.

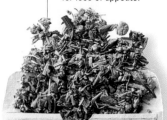

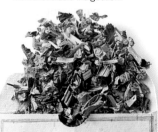

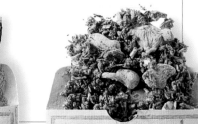

Gentian and mugwort both belong to the group of bitter remedies that stimulate the appetite and improve digestion. They are good at helping to restore digestive function during convalescence. Because of their extremely bitter taste, they are best taken as tinctures in small doses—5 to 10 drops before meals, until appetite returns to normal.

Centaury (*Centaurium umbellatum*) is a bitter and astringent tonic that stimulates the appetite and strengthens the digestive tract in general. It is gentle enough to be given to children, either as a tea—¼ teaspoon centaury in ½ cup boiling water taken before meals—or as a tincture, only for children over five years—5 to 10 drops taken in a little fruit juice two to three times a day before meals. (It is important that children under five who suffer a diminished appetite receive professional medical attention.) Adults should take 10 to 20 drops of centaury three times a day before meals. Its full benefits will be felt after two to three months of treatment.

Horehound is yet another bitter herb that stimulates bile production and can be effective for improving appetite and overcoming indigestion. It has an unpleasant taste and is therefore easier to take as a tincture in small doses—5 drops every hour for acute nausea—rather than as a tea.

ACIDITY OF THE STOMACH AND ULCERS

Too much acid in the stomach can produce symptoms like heartburn after meals. It may also contribute to ulcers forming in the stomach or small intestine. Symptoms of ulcers include stomach pain, indigestion, and regurgitation of food. Although these signs are common and not necessarily serious, if they occur often and for a prolonged period, you should consult a doctor.

Excess stomach acid should be treated with stomachic and demulcent herbs like

---

CAUTION

Take gentian with caution. This bitter root may increase stomach acid and thus exacerbate ulcers. If in doubt, stop treatment and use a gentler remedy or seek the advice of an herbalist. In large doses it can cause headache and nausea.

Vacation herbal first aid

Many people find that a sudden change in diet, alcohol intake, and water quality during their vacation causes stomach disorders. These can range from mild indigestion to serious bouts of diarrhea or constipation. If a stomach upset is caused by an infection, herbal remedies can relieve the symptoms, but the infection must be treated too. Otherwise, a simple herbal first-aid kit that includes a selection of the herbs shown in the column to the right can help to prevent and relieve the various problems caused by vacation stomach upsets.

---

meadowsweet and marsh mallow, which help to regulate the acid content of the stomach. For best effects, they should be taken as tinctures over extended periods of time. Mix meadowsweet and marsh mallow tinctures equally and take 1 teaspoon of the mixture in a little water three times a day before meals. Dietary changes should include cutting out fatty and fried foods, as well as rich, heavy meals. Coffee and alcohol should also be limited.

Licorice has been shown to be an effective aid in the treatment of ulcers, and recent research has confirmed the use of the root as a demulcent and anti-inflammatory remedy. The fresh root yields a thick, sweet juice that should be diluted with hot water and drunk as a tea. It may also be taken as a tincture—1 teaspoon tincture in a little water three times a day—but long-term use should be carefully monitored because licorice can cause water retention and raise blood pressure. Licorice should not be used by people who suffer from high blood pressure.

CONSTIPATION

This is a very common condition and is often caused by a low-fiber diet and lack of exercise. Stressful situations and liver disorders may also contribute, although some people are prone to a lazy bowel and for them constipation may become chronic.

Psyllium (plantain) seeds are a type of bulk-producing laxative. Taken internally they soak up water as they pass through the digestive tract, expanding in volume as they do so. Their bulk stimulates the bowel wall to cause a bowel movement. Psyllium seeds are indigestible and can produce gas, and so are best taken with carminative herbs like fennel or angelica. Sprinkle 1 to 2 teaspoons of psyllium seeds and a pinch

Fennel seeds

Fennel for indigestion and gas

Ginger

Ginger for nausea and vomiting

Peppermint

Peppermint for nausea and gas

Agrimony

Agrimony for diarrhea

Yellow dock

Yellow dock for constipation

Constipation

Constipation is one of the most common health problems in the Western world. Although not a disease in itself, constipation can be a symptom of an underlying condition, or it may be caused by an inappropriate diet, lack of exercise, or nervous tension.

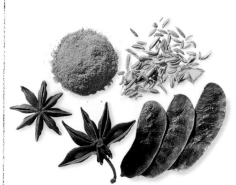

INFUSION FOR CONSTIPATION
Occasionally constipation can be treated with tea or tincture made from fennel, Chinese rhubarb, senna, or star anise.

Some people have difficulty in passing stools or suffer infrequent bowel movements. Either form of chronic constipation may be a natural part of a person's makeup, or it could be a sign of underlying liver problems. In all cases of chronic constipation, it is important that the cause be identified and treated. Very often herbal remedies and simple dietary changes are all that is needed to relieve constipation and keep digestion healthy.

CONSTIPATION BEATERS

It is well established that a low-fiber diet is a major cause of constipation. Fiber is the indigestible part of the food we eat and is found in large amounts in the bran of grains, such as wheat, rye, oats, and barley; legumes, like beans, chickpeas, and lentils; seeds, such as sesame and pumpkin; and fruits and vegetables. Dietary fiber makes up the bulk of stools and stimulates peristalsis, the rhythmic contraction of the bowel walls that moves food through the gut. The more fiber you eat, the more frequent, easy, and complete your bowel movements will become, but you must also increase your fluid intake to soften stools. Drink at least 1 to 2 liters (1 to 2 quarts) of fluid every day. Water is the best choice.

Herbal laxatives
If constipation persists after dietary fiber and exercise have been increased, it may be treated with stimulant laxatives, such as Chinese rhubarb or senna (see page 61 for senna cautions and dosage). Take these before going to bed to produce a bowel movement the next morning. If constipation still continues, seek medical advice. Stimulant laxatives should be avoided during pregnancy and by people who have inflammatory bowel disease or are very weak.

Herbal bulking agents
Plant seeds like psyllium contain large amounts of mucilage and cellulose, which can expand up to three times in volume as they pass through the gut and help make stools larger, softer, and smoother. If you take a bulking agent, make sure you drink at least one glass of liquid at the same time to help it work properly. Taken in this way it will produce a bowel movement in 6 to 12 hours.

BREAKFAST BOOST
Sprinkle 1 to 2 teaspoons of psyllium or crushed flaxseeds on cereal every day. Add a pinch of ground fennel to counteract flatulence.

FIBER IN YOUR DIET
All the fiber you need can be obtained from high-fiber foods.

▶ *Grains—oatmeal, brown rice, whole-grain bread and cereals*
▶ *Legumes— lentils, kidney beans, chickpeas, lima beans, peas*
▶ *Seeds—sesame, sunflower, flax, poppy, pumpkin*
▶ *Fruits—apples, oranges, apricots, peaches, pears, plums, figs*
▶ *Vegetables—celery, carrots, green beans, cabbage, broccoli, potatoes*

of ground fennel on cereal or yogurt and eat this with a cup of herbal tea each evening until the constipation passes.

Stimulant laxatives work by irritating the bowel wall, causing it to contract and expel its contents. Senna, Chinese rhubarb, and aloe belong to this group. Stimulant laxatives can be taken as tinctures but are more effective and kinder to the digestive tract if taken in syrup form: 1 to 2 teaspoons before going to bed will produce a bowel movement in the morning. It is best to combine stimulant laxatives with carminative herbs like fennel or angelica and use them only as a measure of last resort.

DIARRHEA AND COLITIS

Diarrhea can be a sign of an acute infection or the result of a stressful situation or overexcitement. Herbal treatment for diarrhea involves gentle astringent plants to reduce the amount of fluid lost.

Agrimony is a mild but effective remedy that is especially suitable for diarrhea in children. Other helpful herbs include lady's mantle and meadowsweet. These are best taken as a tea—1 cup four times a day—to replace lost fluids. Continue treatment until symptoms pass; if they last for more than two days, consult your doctor.

Colitis is an inflammation of the large intestine that causes alternating diarrhea and constipation and can be very painful. Colitis should always be treated by a doctor. To relieve the symptoms of colitis, agrimony combines well with meadowsweet to make an effective tea; take 1 cup four times a day. Marigold may be added for its anti-inflammatory effect. Studies have shown that agrimony is particularly effective for chronic conditions such as inflammation of the bowel, but the remedies must be taken for at least two to three months.

CAUTION

Stimulant laxatives like senna may cause spasmodic pains and should never be taken by people with inflammatory disease of the bowel (colitis), pregnant women, or anyone who is very weak. If you are unsure about stimulant laxatives, seek advice from a professional herbalist before self-treatment.

Leaves for Digestion

A good way to boost a flagging or weakened digestive system is to increase the herbs in your diet. Herbs with a bitter action promote the production of the stomach juices that serve to break down food. Other herbs have a calming effect and help to settle the stomach after eating. Indigestion can be relieved with carminative herbs. You can use fresh herbs liberally in salads or steam or wilt them in a little hot water and serve them as vegetables.

LIVER AND GALLBLADDER PROBLEMS

Symptoms of liver and gallbladder disease include indigestion, nausea, headaches, constipation, jaundice, and excessive burping, all of which are very common. Often a bad diet rich in fatty foods, excessive alcohol intake, and a generally unhealthy lifestyle can contribute. Both organs can develop serious problems, such as hepatitis or gallstones, so medical advice should be sought if you have any concerns about the seriousness of your condition.

Dandelion, milk thistle, and mugwort are herbs that gently stimulate the liver and gallbladder to produce and secrete enough bile to ensure a healthy digestion. These herbs were included in many old herbal cures, and recent clinical studies have confirmed their claims for therapeutic actions. Roasted dandelion root makes a pleasant drink and should be prepared as a decoction. Drink 1 cup a day as a substitute for coffee.

Milk thistle and mugwort are best taken as tinctures—1 teaspoon two to three times a day with a little water. (Mugwort should be avoided during pregnancy.)

INDIGESTION AND COLIC

The discomfort that occurs after overeating, eating too quickly, or eating the wrong foods is described as indigestion and can be very painful. Herbs like fennel, angelica, and peppermint dispel gas and thus relieve the discomfort of indigestion. For best results, take these herbs as a hot tea; sip 1 cup slowly after meals.

Colic pains are due to intense muscle spasms in the gut, and can be caused by gas or nervous tension. Peppermint is particularly effective for colic pains because of its strongly antispasmodic action. It can be combined with chamomile in a tea, 1 cup taken after each meal.

Angelica

Angelica has a bitter action.

Lemon balm is carminative.

Lemon balm

Dill

Dill helps to calm the stomach.

Dandelion

Dandelion leaf is a bitter herb.

Coriander and Parsley

Coriander has a settling action.

Parsley relieves gas.

RESPIRATORY PROBLEMS

Disorders that restrict breathing, whether they affect the nose, lungs, or airways, can cause serious discomfort. Many herbal remedies can help to relieve and clear congestion.

THYME AND EUCALYPTUS INHALANT Steam inhalations made from thyme and eucalyptus can help to keep the airways clear. Using these herbs as inhalants delivers their antiseptic properties directly to the bronchi. Add 10 drops each of thyme and eucalyptus essential oils to a bowl of hot water and breathe the steam two or three times daily during acute attacks of bronchitis.

A respiratory problem can be caused by an allergic reaction or a viral or bacterial infection. In addition to the discomfort of labored breathing, coughing, and wheezing, such conditions may produce muscular pain, headaches, and dizziness. Herbal remedies can soothe inflamed membranes, clear blocked airways, and relax constricted muscles. A persistent or worsening respiratory disorder should, however, be treated by a doctor.

ASTHMA

Characterized by a tight chest, wheezing, and coughing, asthma is the constriction of bronchial tubes. The condition is caused usually by an allergy to dust, pollen, animal fur, or mold spores, but some cases are triggered by food allergies, and almost all are aggravated by respiratory infections, cold, dry air, exercise, and air pollution. People with asthma should be treated by a doctor.

Herbalists use the Chinese herb ma huang (ephedra) to treat asthma. It has a powerful action that dilates the airways and reduces bronchial spasms. Because of safety concerns for its use, ma huang is not commonly available. (Health Canada warns against products containing ma huang unless they are labeled with a DIN.) The herb has a mild hypertensive action and should not be taken by people with high blood pressure.

Demulcent and antitussive herbs such as marsh mallow, mullein, and coltsfoot help soothe irritated airways and keep them working. Chamomile is particularly useful for childhood asthma if the condition is linked to nervous tension. All these herbs can be taken as tinctures, 1 teaspoon three times a day; teas, 3 cups a day; or syrups, 2 teaspoons three times a day, and should be used over an extended period of time for best results. Children older than five years can take half the adult dose. Do not give these herbal remedies to younger children.

COMMON COLD AND INFLUENZA

The common cold is a viral infection of the upper airways. Symptoms usually include sneezing, a runny nose, general malaise, and sometimes fever. Influenza is an acute viral infection that causes a fever and muscle pain, as well as coughing and a sore throat.

At the first sign of a cold or the flu, take echinacea tincture or plenty of fresh garlic to give your immune system a boost. Both herbs are particularly good at fighting infections in the early stages. Take 2 to 5 ml of echinacea up to four times daily for about a week. There is no limit on your intake of garlic, except that imposed by taste.

BRONCHITIS

An infection of the lower airways, bronchitis is usually indicated by wheezing and coughing up yellow or green phlegm. It may also

Thyme is an excellent expectorant and relaxes bronchial spasms.

Thyme and eucalyptus taken as an inhalation go to work immediately on inflamed bronchi.

Eucalyptus is an antiseptic expectorant that relieves bronchial problems.

THYME AND COLTSFOOT SYRUP

A syrup of thyme and coltsfoot is a very good base to which other herbs may be added as needed, depending on the nature of your cough. A demulcent herb like slippery elm and an expectorant one like mullein will help to relieve a rattling, irritating cough.

Ingredients

1 liter (1 quart) filtered water
55 g (2 oz) dried thyme
55 g (2 oz) dried coltsfoot leaves
  or flowers
450 g (1 lb) granulated sugar

1 *Bring the water to a boil in a stainless-steel saucepan, stir in the dried herbs, and simmer gently over medium heat for 10 minutes.*

2 *Strain the decoction through a clean dish towel or cheesecloth, taking care to squeeze out the residue. Be careful—the herbs may be very hot.*

3 *Transfer the liquid to a heatproof glass or china bowl and place over a small saucepan one-third full of water.*

4 *Bring the water to a boil, lower the heat, and let the decoction reduce slowly down to 250 ml (1⅛ cups). This will take 1 to 2 hours.*

5 *Remove the bowl from the saucepan and add the sugar. Stir the mixture continuously until the sugar has completely dissolved, then leave to cool. When cool, pour into a dark bottle, label, and store in a cool place.*

---

be accompanied by a fever. Herbal treatment of bronchitis concentrates on antitussive and expectorant remedies. Thyme, coltsfoot, and mullein leaf soothe inflamed bronchi and calm excessive coughing. Expectorant herbs like hyssop and elecampane make a cough more productive, so that more phlegm is released and the airways thus freed. The herbs should be taken as syrups or tinctures as short-term remedies; take either 1 teaspoon of tincture or 2 teaspoons of syrup every four hours. Seek medical advice if an attack lasts more than four days.

HAY FEVER

Hay fever, or allergic rhinitis, is an abnormal immune response to flowers, grass, or tree pollen. Symptoms include sneezing, a runny nose, itchy, swollen eyes, and breathing difficulties, and can last from spring to early autumn.

Elderflower, plantain, and eyebright have a tonic effect on the lining of the nose and throat and help them resist seasonal attacks from pollen. Hay fever remedies should be taken either as teas or tinctures in standard doses. For best results, they must be used throughout the year, not just at dangerous times or during attacks.

Chinese herbalists use the herb ma huang to treat acute attacks of hay fever because of its antiallergic properties. Nettle also has antiallergic properties and may safely be used instead of ma huang, which is not commonly available. Drink 1 cup of nettle tea up to four times a day.

An infusion made from peppermint, elderflower, yarrow, and ginger will ease the worst symptoms of a cold and relieve the aches and pains of flu. To benefit from its warming and diaphoretic qualities, you should sip 3 to 4 cups of hot brew a day.

A bath containing essential oils will also help sweat out a cold, but should not be used in feverish conditions. Add a few drops of rosemary, eucalyptus, or peppermint essential oils to a hot bath.

COUGH

A cough is the body's attempt to clear the lungs and bronchi of irritants or excess mucus. It can be a sign of an infection, such as bronchitis, or it may be a symptom of hay fever or nervous tension.

For a rattling cough, use expectorant herbs to help the airways expel excess phlegm. Choose herbs that also have demulcent properties to soothe any irritation. Good expectorant herbs are mullein, elecampane, coltsfoot, angelica, and hyssop. Mullein and coltsfoot combined have both demulcent and expectorant properties. Cough medicines are best taken as syrups because they soothe the inflamed airways and are easy to make at home (see above).

To relax the airways, choose thyme or hyssop, and for a chesty cough, add an expectorant herb such as elecampane. Add 20 ml (4 teaspoons) of tincture to 100 ml (3½ fl oz) of syrup base. Adults can take 10 ml (2 teaspoons) 3 to 4 times a day; children should take 5 ml (1 teaspoon) 3 to 4 times a day.

REPRODUCTIVE AND URINARY PROBLEMS

Reproductive and urinary disorders can be both distressing and embarrassing. Herbal remedies can help not only to relieve symptoms but also reduce the frequency of urogenital problems.

HERBS AND

MENSTRUAL PROBLEMS
Shepherd's purse and lady's mantle help reduce excessive bleeding. They may be taken as a tea or tincture, individually or in combination.

For cramping pains that occur before a period starts or during the first two days, cramp bark tincture can be helpful. Take up to 3 teaspoons in warm water three times a day for acute pains. Hot chamomile tea, sipped slowly throughout the day, also soothes menstrual pain and helps to relieve any accompanying tension.

The majority of herbal remedies that offer relief from reproductive and urinary problems are taken internally as teas or tinctures, but some, such as those with antifungal properties, can be applied topically in ointments and creams.

PREMENSTRUAL SYNDROME (PMS)
Hormonal changes in the days leading up to a period can cause depression, irritability, anxiety, tenderness of the breasts, and water retention. The severity and occurrence of these symptoms vary among individuals.

One of the most highly favored herbs for premenstrual syndrome is chasteberry (*Vitex agnus-castus*). It has long been used to treat gynecological problems, and British studies have confirmed that it is particularly effective at relieving such physical symptoms of PMS as water retention and tender breasts. To achieve the best results, take 20 drops of chasteberry tincture every morning for at least six months.

Evening primrose oil, available in capsules, is also highly recommended for PMS. For emotional ups and downs, drink teas of gentle, relaxing herbs such as chamomile and lemon balm throughout the month. Take 1 to 2 cups daily and 3 to 4 cups in the days leading up to your period.

MENOPAUSAL PROBLEMS
For months or even years before menopause, a woman may experience both physical and emotional changes due to hormonal changes in the body. Chasteberry—¼ teaspoon of crushed dried fruit or 1 to 2 teaspoons of standardized extract each day—can help regulate these changes. To ease stress, a combined infusion of motherwort and lemon balm can be used each day. Herbs that help counter hot flashes include licorice (*Glycyrrhiza glabra*), sage (*salvia officinalis*), and black cohosh (*Cimicifuga racemosa*). The first two are effective as teas; the last one can be taken as a tincture—1 teaspoon twice a day—or an extract—½ teaspoon daily.

Research has recently been conducted into the hormone-regulating properties of *Rheum rhaponticum*, a species of rhubarb. The root of the plant is thought to have an estrogenic action. However, studies have not yet been conclusive and further research is being done.

SEXUAL IMPOTENCE
Impotence may be due to stress and nervous tension or caused by a physical problem such as prostatitis (inflammation of the prostate gland). Certain conventional drugs have also been found to reduce a man's ability to achieve or sustain an erection.

Some herbal tonics like damiana and saw palmetto do have a specific action on the male reproductive system. Others have an

Lady's mantle helps to reduce the pain of heavy periods.

Shepherd's purse can help ease excessive bleeding.

Shepherd's purse and lady's mantle tea can be sipped every few hours during painful periods.

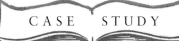

CASE STUDY

A Woman with Painful Periods

Most women suffer from menstrual pain at some time in their lives. Although the possible causes are numerous, they often include stress, poor eating habits, and lack of sufficient exercise. For many the pain is only mildly uncomfortable, but others suffer greatly. Fortunately, many menstrual problems respond well to natural herbal remedies.

Julie, a landscape gardener, is 26 and single. She greatly enjoys her job and is a lively, outgoing person with an active social life. Unfortunately, the pace of her life means she sometimes misses meals. For years Julie has had menstrual problems; her periods tend to be very heavy, with painful abdominal cramps two days before bleeding starts. She usually copes, but has had to take time off from work sometimes because the pain is so bad. It is eased with over-the-counter painkillers, but they do not relieve the nausea she often feels. Adding to her frustration, Julie has never had a regular menstrual cycle. Her doctor advised her to take oral contraceptives to regulate the periods and reduce the pain, but Julie is reluctant to do so.

WHAT JULIE SHOULD DO

Julie has had painful periods for so long they are likely caused by hormonal imbalance. To regulate her hormone levels, Julie can take 15 to 20 drops of chasteberry tincture every morning before breakfast. Chasteberry is slow-acting and must be taken for at least six months before improvements will show.

Julie might also take herbal tonics to improve the general health of her uterus and ovaries. Herbs like marigold and lady's mantle are good tonics and can be taken as tinctures.

Evening primrose oil capsules will ease symptoms of premenstrual syndrome. Drinking a cup of ginger and chamomile tea four times a day in the days preceding her period should relieve Julie's nausea and pain.

Action Plan

DIET
Increase intake of iron-rich foods, including green leafy vegetables, seafood, and legumes. Cut back on salty foods (to reduce water retention) and caffeine.

LIFESTYLE
Take time to relax and unwind. Find a meditation class or go for long walks to release tension.

HEALTH
Herbal treatments can help relieve painful menstrual periods, as well as aid relaxation. Julie should also talk to her doctor about taking vitamin and mineral supplements.

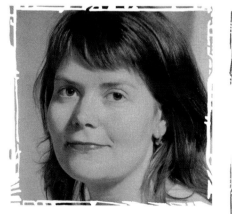

HEALTH
Constant use of painkillers may increase fatigue and cause side effects such as nausea and iron deficiency.

DIET
A lack of regular nutrient-rich foods can cause the body to respond badly to pain and extend recovery time.

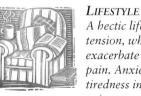

LIFESTYLE
A hectic life can cause tension, which may exacerbate menstrual pain. Anxiety and tiredness increase pain response.

HOW THINGS TURNED OUT FOR JULIE

After four months of herbal treatment, Julie's periods are less painful but she still has cramps on the day before her period starts. She finds that the herbal tea stops the nausea and takes away the worst of the pain. Her menstrual cycle is still irregular, but she has noticed sufficient signs of improvement, which make her determined to continue the treatment, maintain her better eating habits, and learn more about stress reduction.

indirect action, strengthening the body as a whole; these include ginseng and other nerve tonics, such as oats and skullcap. Studies are being done to determine ginkgo biloba's circulatory action in relation to the reproductive organs. To be effective, all these herbs must be taken long-term as teas, capsules, or tinctures in standard doses.

INFERTILITY

Infertility can be due to a number of causes, and the majority of them usually require long-term treatment. Any approach should be carried out under professional supervision. Infertility caused by a hormone imbalance may respond well to chasteberry taken every morning for at least six months.

Herbs that help keep the female reproductive system healthy include marigold, lady's mantle, and raspberry leaf. Marigold is beneficial for any underlying chronic inflammation of the reproductive system. Lady's mantle and raspberry leaf are traditional tonic herbs that strengthen the womb and ovaries. All of these herbs can be taken every day as a tincture or as a tea.

CANDIDIASIS

A fungal infection caused by *Candida albicans*, candidiasis most commonly affects the vagina, causing itchy red skin and a cloudy white discharge. To treat the condition, use immune-stimulating herbs like garlic, echinacea, and marigold. These are best taken in tincture form—1 teaspoon up to four times a day for acute attacks. In addition, cleavers and marigold tea can be taken long-term to improve lymphatic drainage and thus help the immune system deal with the infection.

You can combine internal treatment with external applications of antifungal herbs. Tea tree and thyme essential oils have strong antifungal properties. Add 15 to 20 drops of each to 25 g (1 fl oz) of base cream and apply twice daily for as long as the symptoms persist. Infused oil of marigold will reduce redness and irritation. A low-sugar diet will also help fight the problem.

CYSTITIS

A common condition that affects primarily women, cystitis has symptoms that include an urgency to pass water, burning pain on urination, and sometimes blood in the urine.

Herbs like juniper, plantain, and yarrow are traditional remedies for urinary infections. They have a mild antiseptic action on the bladder and should be combined with demulcent herbs such as marsh mallow and diuretics like dandelion leaf, which will help to reduce the pain.

Take cystitis remedies as a tea—1 cup every four hours—to help flush out the bladder. Make sure you continue the course of treatment until all symptoms have disappeared. Use juniper with caution. It has a strong irritant action on the kidneys and should not be used by people who have a kidney condition or are pregnant.

PROSTATE ENLARGEMENT

A common condition in men over 40 years of age, enlargement of the prostate develops slowly and is characterized by an increasing difficulty and need to urinate. These symptoms should be checked by a doctor to exclude cancer of the prostate.

Saw palmetto, nettle, and horsetail are recommended in traditional and modern herbal medicine for an enlarged prostate. Nettle root has been shown to be particularly beneficial in the early stages of prostate problems. For best results, nettle root should be taken as a tincture or prepared as a decoction, both taken in standard doses for long-term use.

Herbal Myths

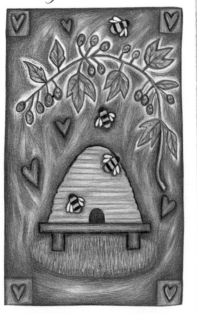

Hops that have been infused in boiling water, strained, and mixed with honey make a simple modern equivalent of an ancient Teutonic female aphrodisiac known as honey-beer. New brides of ancient times would drink a mixture of fermented hops and honey each day for 30 days after their wedding ceremony to heighten their sexual responsiveness and increase their pleasure. This custom led to the term honeymoon. "Moon" is an archaic and poetic term that means a month.

HAIR AND SKIN PROBLEMS

Many health problems—from acne to dandruff—can affect your skin and hair. The majority can be relieved and treated with readily available, simple, and effective herbal remedies.

As the outside protective layer of the body, the skin is particularly susceptible to injury and infection. It is also true that healthy skin and hair reflect the overall health of the body and are useful diagnostic tools for doctors.

BRUISING
A blow to the skin can damage the capillaries beneath the surface, causing discoloration as blood spreads into the tissues. The discoloration varies, turning blue, green, brown, purple, and yellow as the bruise heals. Most bruises are tender to the touch and are accompanied by swelling.

Prompt treatment can minimize swelling and discoloration. A witch hazel compress is an excellent first-aid treatment for a bruise. If bruising is accompanied by swelling and the skin feels very hot, a compress soaked in two parts witch hazel and one part cider vinegar will help. Compresses should cover the whole affected area and be changed frequently. A compress of arnica (1 part tincture with 3 to 10 parts water) may also reduce inflammation and swelling.

BURNS
Superficial burns with reddened skin and slight blistering may be treated at home. More serious and extensive burns must receive prompt medical attention. Burns should be treated straightaway with cold running water until the skin has cooled to normal temperature, then a few drops of lavender essential oil can be applied directly to the burn. This will help to keep the skin clean, reduce the pain, and speed the healing process. Once the immediate trauma is over, anti-inflammatory herbs like marigold and St. John's wort will help the burn to

heal speedily. They may be used as creams or infused oils, applied liberally three or four times a day. Aloe vera gel can also help; it is cooling and anti-inflammatory.

CUTS AND GRAZES
Small cuts and grazes are easily treated at home, but deep wounds should be checked by a doctor to prevent infection.

A number of herbs are used to treat superficial wounds. Diluted marigold tincture has known antiseptic and anti-inflammatory properties and is useful for cleaning a dirty

MAKING AN HERBAL SKIN SPRAY

Some skin conditions may be too painful to touch, which can make applying remedies an ordeal. A spray bottle allows you to apply herbal remedies directly without exacerbating problems. It is good especially for soothing and cooling painful sunburn.

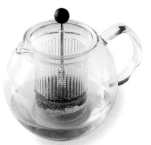

1 *Make an infusion or decoction of cooling or anti-inflammatory herbs, such as marigold, lavender, chamomile, or lime flowers.*

2 *Pour the cooled liquid into a clean spray bottle and secure the lid.*

3 *Spray a light film of the preparation over the affected area and allow to evaporate.*

cut to prevent it from becoming infected. Echinacea tincture may be used in the same way. Dilute one part of tincture with three parts of water and use a sterile dressing pad to clean the cut and surrounding skin.

Inflamed and slow-healing wounds can be treated with comfrey, marigold, or calendula ointment. Many studies have confirmed the use of these herbs as wound-healing remedies. Comfrey, in particular, is effective on slow-healing cuts and grazes and is known to lessen scar formation. However, it must never be applied to large areas of broken skin because it is toxic.

WARTS AND CORNS

Warts are small, hard, and uneven lesions that form on the skin, often of the hands and feet; they are caused by a virus. Traditionally, the fresh juice of dandelion flower stalks was used to treat warts. It was applied directly over the wart to seal it until it disappeared. Slices of fresh garlic are also a traditional remedy. Apply for several minutes once a day until the wart disappears.

Corns, thickened areas on the feet, are usually caused by ill-fitting shoes that put pressure on the skin, especially around the toes. The skin grows very thick, and continued friction may make it inflamed and sore.

A cream with infused oil of marigold and essential oil of chamomile can help to soothe red and inflamed feet. Massage the cream into your feet daily. Both herbs have excellent anti-inflammatory and wound-healing properties. For very thick corns, massage marigold oil ointment well into the skin every day. Ointments keep the skin soft and are good for use on small patches.

SORE FEET
Prolonged spells of standing or walking, especially in ill-fitting shoes, can cause sore feet. The skin may develop painful blisters as well. Essential oil of peppermint added to cool water (see below) will have a soothing action on the skin. A strong infusion of peppermint, allowed to cool, is an effective footbath also. Afterward, massage your feet gently with marigold or chamomile cream, taking care not to burst any blisters.

Peppermint foot cream

Peppermint cream or a mint footbath can quickly relieve the pain of tired, sore feet. For a bath, add 5 drops of peppermint oil to a bowl of cold water and soak your feet in it for 10 minutes. This will cool and refresh them.

Mint

ATHLETE'S FOOT

Athlete's foot is a common fungal infection of the feet. The microbes that cause fungal infections thrive in warm, sweaty conditions such as those common in closed shoes and boots, and poor hygiene makes the problem worse. The condition is notoriously difficult to treat and requires both internal and external remedies.

Two to three cups of cleavers or marigold tea taken daily will help to improve lymphatic drainage and rid the body of fungal infections. Increasing fresh garlic in the diet can also be beneficial.

Externally, antifungal herbs like garlic, goldenseal, marigold, and essential oil of tea tree or thyme should be applied daily. The tinctures can be used undiluted on the skin or mixed into a base cream. Scrupulous hygiene is also essential, and feet must be dried thoroughly after washing and before treatments are applied. Although goldenseal must not be used internally by pregnant women, it is completely safe to use externally in combination with other herbs.

PSORIASIS

Psoriasis occurs when skin cells overproduce, causing patches of red, scaly, itchy skin. The exact causes are unknown, but attacks can be triggered by stress, and susceptibility to psoriasis often runs in families. Psoriasis is very common and can be severe.

The internal treatment of psoriasis is similar to that of eczema (see below), involving alterative or nervine herbs, depending on which is appropriate. Evening primrose oil, taken internally as capsules, often helps to improve the elasticity of the skin and reduce the extent of dry and flaky skin patches.

External herbal preparations should be rich and oily to moisturize the skin and reduce flakiness. Small patches of psoriasis can be treated with marigold, chickweed, or marsh mallow ointment to protect and soothe the skin. For large areas of psoriasis, use infused oils of marigold, chickweed, or even plain olive oil. Add peppermint if the skin is very itchy.

ECZEMA

The symptoms of eczema are red and sore patches on the skin, often in the crook of the elbow, behind the knees, or on the hands. The affected skin can also become wet, weepy, and extremely itchy. Some forms of

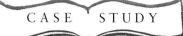

A Psoriasis Sufferer

Psoriasis, characterized by patches of red, itchy, and scaly skin, is one of the most common skin diseases in the Western world, affecting up to 2 percent of people. Despite intensive research, it remains difficult to treat. However, herbs and dietary changes can help to relieve the symptoms and reduce the frequency of attacks.

Jane is a 35-year-old teacher. She has had sensitive skin since childhood, but recently she began to develop small patches of red, scaly skin on her elbows. Initially Jane paid little attention, particularly because she noticed that they always cleared up during her vacation. When her long-term relationship ended, however, her skin condition suddenly exploded, and the rash now covers her arms entirely.

Worried, Jane visited her doctor, who diagnosed psoriasis and prescribed medicated creams but explained that they would not prevent the rash from recurring. The doctor also referred Jane to a clinic for ultraviolet treatment, because judicious exposure to the UVB rays of the sun is beneficial to psoriasis.

WHAT JANE SHOULD DO
Jane should make sure that her diet contains plenty of sunflower or canola oil. These contain a high percentage of polyunsaturated fatty acids, which are important for a healthy skin. A friend at work advised Jane to visit an herbalist, who recommended evening primrose oil capsules. The herbalist also tried to balance Jane's metabolism and improve her overall health with gentle bitters, diuretics, and alterative herbs, including nettle, dandelion root and leaf, and figwort. Jane should expect her condition to become worse initially as her metabolism adjusts. A rich cream made from infused oils of marigold and cleavers applied daily will help relieve the itching.

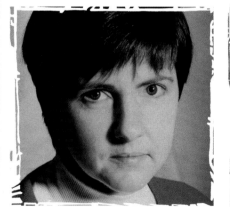

EMOTIONAL HEALTH
Emotional distress can worsen psoriasis. Underlying problems must be addressed as part of the treatment.

LIFESTYLE
Sunshine and seawater are beneficial for psoriasis and will help relieve the immediate symptoms. Dietary changes will also help.

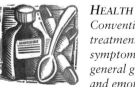

HEALTH
Conventional treatments can relieve symptoms, but general good physical and emotional health is the best way to help to stave off the triggers of psoriasis attacks.

Action Plan

DIET
Consume more coldwater fish, also flaxseed oil, for their omega 3 fatty acids. Eat less meat and other animal foods and more yellow fruits and vegetables and leafy greens for vitamins A and C.

LIFESTYLE
Choose the seaside for your next vacation if you can. Sunshine, swimming, and long walks on the beach will help your skin recover.

HEALTH
See an herbalist to discuss a holistic approach, addressing stress and emotional problems especially.

HOW THINGS TURNED OUT FOR JANE

After the first two weeks of herbal treatment, Jane's skin became very red and itchy. Jane found this difficult to cope with, but drinking lime flower tea, in addition to her prescribed herbal medicines, helped her with the emotional distress. Jane also discovered that she needed to apply the cream frequently at first, up to five times a day, to get relief. Two months after the initial treatment, Jane's condition is finally improving.

Hair loss treatments

The best herbal treatments are hair lotions that stimulate blood flow to the scalp and the roots of the hair. Increased circulation provides the hair with nutrients that help it to grow.

A traditional recipe for a hair lotion includes 1 ml (20 drops) of rosemary essential oil, 1 ml (20 drops) of lavender essential oil, and 30 ml (2 tablespoons) of nettle tincture mixed with 75 ml (⅓ cup) of water. Massage well into the scalp at night. This lotion may be used long-term.

eczema are allergic reactions; others may be genetic, although both are notoriously difficult to treat. The underlying cause should be identified and treated whenever possible. Herbal medicine for the skin always combines external preparations with internal treatment. Traditional herbal remedies are alteratives like burdock, cleavers, figwort, and nettle, which improve the general health of the body. If eczema is associated with nervous tension, nervines—nerve relaxants such as oats and lime flowers—should also be included. Herbal treatment for eczema is always long-term, and the herbs may be taken as teas or tinctures, using standard doses.

Herbs like chickweed, marigold, and burdock can be used externally to soothe the irritation. Peppermint may be added if the skin is very itchy. The herbs can be made into creams or be used as infused oils and applied to the affected parts several times a day. For very weepy eczema, make a strong tea from walnut leaves and apply this as a compress twice a day. Let the skin dry naturally, and then apply a light marigold or chickweed cream.

DANDRUFF

In this itchy condition of the scalp, the top layer of the skin sheds its dead cells at a faster rate than normal. The old skin is seen as white flakes in the hair and usually on the sufferer's clothes.

Many skin problems are a sign that the body is not in the best of health. In some cases, too much junk food and a lack of sufficient vitamins and polyunsaturated oils in the diet contribute to the problem.

Internal herbal treatment should include bitter herbs like dandelion or gentian to encourage elimination of toxins. Herbalists also include alterative herbs such as nettle and burdock. A good combination is a tincture made from equal parts of dandelion leaf and root, nettle, and figwort, taken in standard doses over long periods.

For immediate improvement, while waiting for internal treatments to take effect, mix together 30 drops each of sandalwood and rosemary essential oils with 60 ml (¼ cup) almond oil. Shake well and massage into the scalp. Leave for half an hour, then shampoo. Repeat this routine every time you wash your hair, and be sure to rinse your hair thoroughly after using the oils to remove any loosened skin cells.

HAIR LOSS

Hair constantly regenerates itself, and losing a small amount is normal. Abnormal hair loss, however, may be due to poor general health, stress, or genetic factors.

Unfortunately, if hair loss is hereditary, there are few herbal treatments that will be of use. For hair loss that is due to poor health or stress, herbalism can offer some help (see far left column).

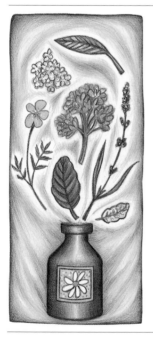

HERBS FOR YOUR HAIR TYPE

Herbs can have a dramatic effect on the health of your hair. Some preparations help control common problems such as dandruff, while others enhance the natural color of your hair. Specific hair conditions, such as blonde hair being particularly fine, can also be improved with a selection of herbal hair rinses.

HAIR TYPE	SUGGESTED HERBS
Fair	Chamomile, calendula, elderflower, mullein, rhubarb root (powdered), saffron, turmeric, yarrow
Dark	Comfrey, marjoram, nettle, parsley, raspberry leaf, rosemary, sage, southernwood, thyme
Red	Marigold flowers, red hibiscus, red oak bark (ground to a powder), ginger, saffron
Gray	Betony, marjoram, nettle, rosemary, sage, walnut
Oily	Geranium, lavender, lemon balm, parsley, peppermint, rosemary, white dead nettle, witch hazel
Dry	Burdock root, calendula, chamomile, comfrey, elde flower, lavender, marsh mallow, sandalwood
Dull	Calendula, fennel leaf, parsley, rosemary, southernwood, stinging nettle
Dandruff	Basil, burdock root, cleavers, cypress, lavender, mint, nettle, parsley, rosemary, southernwood
Thinning	Bay, chamomile, cedarwood, clary sage, cypress, horsetail (stems and branches), southernwood

EAR AND EYE PROBLEMS

Any loss of hearing or impairment of vision must be treated by your doctor. Some milder disorders, however, respond well to herbal remedies.

Ailments of the ears and eyes can be highly disturbing and painful, and some simple problems can have more vexing side effects. An earache, for example, can cause balance problems, while inflammation of the eyelids can affect vision as the eyelids swell.

ACUTE EARACHE

Acute earache is usually a symptom of an infection of the middle ear or the ear canal. Such infections need to be treated internally with immune-stimulating herbs like echinacea, goldenseal, or garlic. Take 1 teaspoon of tincture up to four times a day until the infection has cleared. (Goldenseal, which stimulates the muscles of the uterus, should not be taken by pregnant women.)

CHRONIC EARACHE

Some people have very sensitive ears that become painful during cold and windy weather. Chronic earache may also be caused by catarrh in the middle ear, which must be treated with anticatarrhal herbs like elderflower and eyebright. A tincture of the herbs should be taken over several months.

Mullein oil or plain olive oil may be used for chronic earache. Use a few drops of the warm oil (see box, right) in the ear canal during cold weather to protect the eardrum.

CONJUNCTIVITIS

Inflammation of the conjunctiva, the delicate lining of the eye, causes redness, itching, and weeping. This inflammation may be due to hay fever, irritation from dust or sand, or an infection. Conjunctivitis responds well to external treatment with herbal remedies. Combine eyebright and fennel and make a strong infusion. Strain this well before use to prevent further irritation of the eye. Add a pinch of salt and use as an eye lotion, gently bathing the eyelid several times a day with a pad of cotton soaked in the mixture, until the condition has improved.

INFLAMMATION OF THE EYELIDS

Allergies or infections that affect the eyelids may cause conjunctivitis-like symptoms, but there is usually pus around the eyelid, which becomes very tender as a result.

Applying warm compresses soaked in a strong infusion of chamomile is one effective treatment. Chamomile has a strong anti-inflammatory action on the skin, and various studies have found it to be both antiseptic and analgesic. Treat the infected eyelid frequently throughout the day with chamomile compresses until the condition has improved.

HOMEMADE EAR DROPS

To relieve earache, use a few drops of infused oil of mullein flowers in the ear. Add 1 drop of essential oil of clove if the pain is severe. Never use external remedies on a perforated eardrum; if in doubt, consult your doctor before self-treatment.

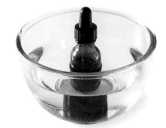

1 *Put oil in a bottle that has a dropper; stand it in a bowl of warm water for 10 to 15 minutes.*

2 *Put 2 to 3 drops of the warm oil in each ear and seal with cotton balls. Repeat two or three times a day.*

MOUTH, TEETH, AND THROAT PROBLEMS

Herbal remedies can offer effective relief from a variety of disorders affecting the mouth, teeth, and throat. These range from catarrhal bad breath to mouth ulcers to a sore throat.

Mouth ulcers and toothache are common problems that can be relieved with herbs. While acute infections of the throat can also be treated with herbs, chronic ailments, which may be symptoms of allergies or more serious underlying disorders, should be properly diagnosed before herbal treatment is applied.

BLEEDING GUMS

Sore and bleeding gums are signs of gum disease. Gingivitis, or inflammation of the gums, is one of the most common infections of the mouth. It may be caused by poor oral hygiene and a high-sugar diet.

Sage is the most popular herb for treating bleeding gums because of its astringent and antibacterial properties. Studies in Germany have confirmed its effectiveness for the treatment of bacterial and viral infections in the mouth, including gingivitis. A strong infusion of sage can be used as a mouthwash three times a day for as long as the infection persists. Other astringent herbs used in this way include a decoction of marigold flowers and witch hazel bark.

COLD SORES

The small weeping blisters on the lips known as cold sores are caused by the herpes simplex virus. An attack may be triggered when the body's resistance is low, for instance, during infection with a cold or at times of high or prolonged stress.

Cold sores must be treated both internally and externally. Herbs to boost the immune system, such as echinacea and St. John's wort, should be taken at the first sign of a blister—5 milliliters of tincture three times a day—until the infection passes.

A cream made with essential oil of lemon balm and infused oil of St. John's wort will help heal a cold sore externally. Studies on lemon balm have confirmed antiviral properties. Apply the cream frequently throughout the day until the infection has cleared.

TOOTHACHE

A symptom of tooth decay, toothache must be treated by a dentist. However, herbs can help relieve the pain. A traditional treatment is to crack a clove between the teeth, then hold it between the affected gum and the cheek; or apply a cotton ball soaked in clove oil to the painful tooth and leave it until the pain subsides (see page 45).

Another approach is to apply a fresh slice of ginger to the affected area and leave until the burning becomes intolerable; or soak a cotton ball in water, squeeze out the excess, apply 2 to 4 drops of thyme oil, and hold it against the aching gum for a few minutes.

BAD BREATH (HALITOSIS)
Although bad breath can be overpowering and embarrassing, it is easily treatable. It may be a sign of poor oral hygiene, digestive problems, bad diet, or an infection of the mouth or throat.

Angelica

Marigold

Chew aromatic herbs like angelica and parsley to freshen the breath. See a dentist for a thorough cleaning of gums and teeth.

Use astringent herbs like sage and marigold to treat gingivitis. Infections of the gums, mouth, and throat can lead to halitosis.

Parsley

Eat bitter herbs such as dandelion to keep the digestive system healthy. Digestive disorders and a high-sugar diet may worsen breath problems.

Sage

Dandelion

SAGE VINEGAR FOR A SORE THROAT

Macerating herbs in vinegar for medicinal use is an old folk tradition. This remedy for sore throats combines the astringent and antiseptic properties of sage with the anti-inflammatory action of vinegar.

Dilute one part sage vinegar with two parts water, add a pinch of salt, and gargle with it three times a day until the condition improves. Alternatively, soak a clean handkerchief in the solution and wring out the excess. Wrap the compress around your throat and cover with a clean towel. Renew after 15 minutes. Repeat three times a day.

Ingredients
2 large sprigs fresh sage
    or 1 tbsp dried sage
425 ml (1¾ cups) cider vinegar

1 *If you are using fresh sage, remove the leaves from the stems and chop them coarsely in order to release the active ingredients. If using dried sage, crumble the leaves slightly. Put the sage in a one-pint glass jar that has a tight-fitting lid.*

2 *In a glass or stainless-steel saucepan, gently heat the cider vinegar over low heat until it reaches body temperature. Pour it over the sage, seal the jar, and shake well.*

3 *Leave on a sunny windowsill for two weeks, shaking the jar vigorously every day. Strain the liquid into a sterilized glass bottle and stopper well. Label and date. Stored in a cool, dark place, it will keep for up to one year.*

DENTAL PLAQUE

A buildup of dental plaque is the result of poor oral hygiene. Dental plaque encourages the growth of the bacteria that cause tooth decay. You can look for a toothpaste that contains astringent and anti-inflammatory herbs such as sage, peppermint, chamomile, or echinacea. The addition of salt or bicarbonate of soda makes a toothpaste mildly abrasive, which helps reduce plaque.

MOUTH ULCERS

Painful mouth ulcers are a sign of a low immune system and commonly occur after a cold or during emotionally stressful periods. Marigold and myrrh are popular remedies. Herbal practice has shown them to be very effective, possibly because of their antiseptic and anti-inflammatory properties. Dilute their tinctures in water (1 part tincture to 4 parts water) and use as a mouthwash three times a day until the ulcers have cleared.

Herbs like echinacea that stimulate the immune system should be taken internally. Take a capsule or 1 teaspoon of tincture up to four times a day until the ulcers clear up.

SORE THROAT

A sore throat is a very annoying condition; it can be caused by a virus (usually at the start of a cold) or by a bacterial infection, which is usually more serious. The throat feels very hot, and swallowing can be difficult. Herbal treatment for sore throats, consisting of gargles and compresses, can be highly effective. If a sore throat is severe and lasts for more than three days, you should consult a doctor rather than continue self-treatment. If, however, it is only a mild sore throat, accompanying a cold, for example, then the following herbal preparations may help to speed recovery.

A demulcent herb like marsh mallow makes a very effective, soothing remedy. A cold infusion made from the leaves of the plant should be used as a gargle three to four times a day until the condition has improved. Add astringent and antiseptic herbs like sage, myrrh, and marigold to heal the underlying infection.

Drink sage or marigold tea to soothe any inflammation and to help your tonsils to recover from infection. You can use the tea as a gargle and drink a cup of the infusion three times a day until the infection clears.

Cider vinegar compresses are an old folk remedy for sore throats. Add one part of vinegar to three parts of lukewarm water and apply externally as a compress. Repeat the treatment three times a day until your condition improves.

Vinegar compresses will help draw out heat and reduce inflammation in your throat. They are useful if the throat feels very hot, tender, and swollen. Use a compress in addition to gargling if possible. The joint treatment should help to relieve the pain of a sore throat very quickly.

149

MIGRAINES AND OTHER HEADACHES

Muscular tension, eyestrain, and allergic reactions can all be responsible for headaches. Herbal remedies offer relief from the pain and nausea that may accompany them.

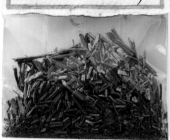

Vervain compress
For quick and gentle relief from a mild vascular headache, make a cold compress with an infusion of vervain and apply it to the forehead and back of the neck until the headache clears.

Mankind has long suffered from headaches, and herbalism has offered many remedies for them. Although in general headaches are a response to physical or emotional stress, most arise from just two basic causes—tension and vascular disturbances. Headaches are usually no cause for worry, but if they are chronic or severe, you should see a doctor.

HEADACHE
Headaches caused by nervous tension rarely follow a recognizable symptom pattern, although there is usually muscle tension in the shoulders and neck. Relaxing and calming herbs can be used both internally and externally to treat tension headaches.

Gentle relaxants such as lemon balm, chamomile, and valerian make useful remedies because of their sedative and antispasmodic properties. They are best when taken as teas and can be drunk throughout the day. One cup at night will also aid sleep.

The essential oils of lavender and peppermint have a mild sedative action. Dab a small amount on each temple and on your forehead, rub it in gently, and remain quiet for several minutes. Lavender oil is also effective when used in an essential oil burner or a warm bath. Warm water enhances its relaxing effect on muscles and the nervous system. Use lavender oil sparingly in a bath, adding no more than 10 drops; large doses may have the opposite effect.

Headaches that are triggered by food or drink can also be relieved with the relaxant and mildly sedative herbs mentioned above.

MIGRAINE
Migraine headaches, caused by disturbances in the vascular system, are often accompanied by nausea, vomiting, and sensitivity to light. Attacks can last for hours, even days.

Factors that can trigger a migraine are numerous and include foods such as cheese and chocolate, weather changes, and stress. In all cases the cause of the underlying problem should be identified before any long-term treatment is decided upon.

Feverfew is excellent for migraine because it relaxes and dilates the blood vessels in the head, which contract during an attack and cause pain. It is best to take the fresh herb on a regular basis as a preventive measure. You can do this by eating three or four leaves with a little bread. If the leaves irritate your mouth, take a tincture of the herb—5 millileters every day—or try feverfew capsules. Feverfew has a stimulant action on the uterus and must not be taken by women during pregnancy.

Plants that contain caffeine, like coffee, tea, and kola nut, can help check acute migraines. Although excessive doses of caffeine may actually trigger a migraine, small amounts are valuable for treating severe attacks because they constrict blood vessels.

Pathway to health
Headaches brought on by stress or tension can be relieved with herbal remedies that soothe the tension behind the pain. You can enhance the beneficial effect of the herbs by practicing relaxation and visualization techniques, such as picturing yourself floating in warm water. The dual assault on the tension will quickly ease your headache.

MUSCLE PAIN

Aching muscles are a familiar symptom of strenuous exercise, bad posture, and influenza. Herbal remedies can help to relieve pain and ease muscular tension.

Muscles can become painful as a result of overexertion, which will cause tiny tears and inflammation in the muscle tissue. These tears usually take two to three days to heal, but herbal oils and creams applied externally can soothe the pain and speed recovery.

Touch is a powerful healing tool, and using herbal oils to massage away tension is a very effective way of relieving the discomfort of aching muscles. External treatment in the form of massage oils, creams, hot compresses, and baths is best for muscular pain. Infused oils made from rubefacient herbs like mustard or cayenne pepper also make very good massage oils or can be added to a base cream. Alternatively, essential oils and an infused oil can be combined to enhance and tailor their effects.

BEFORE A MASSAGE

To prepare muscles for massage treatment, take a warm bath, which will relax and loosen them. It is easier to apply a cream or massage oil if the skin is supple and the muscles are relaxed. You can add essential oils of invigorating herbs such as rosemary, thyme, or eucalyptus to the bathwater to stimulate circulation.

If you do not have time for a bath or just want to relieve aches and pains in your legs, soak your feet in a hot footbath instead. Fill a deep bowl or bucket with warm water (just above body temperature is ideal), add 5 drops of an essential oil such as thyme or rosemary, and soak your feet for 10 to 15 minutes. This will stimulate blood flow to the legs and feet and make the absorption of oils and creams easier. A footbath is also a

TYPES OF MUSCLE PAIN AND REMEDIES

Whatever the cause of your muscle pain, there are herbal strategies to help. To make your own remedy for aching muscles, choose essential oils of herbs from the following categories. If your muscle pains are accompanied by tenderness and swelling, try using cooling herbs like peppermint to hasten the healing process. Use the essential oil on a compress or in a cream, or add it to a base oil and massage gently into the skin. If muscles ache because of a cold or bout of flu, gentle massage with herbal oils will ease these muscular aches until time restores you to health. If a muscle cramp is the problem, it can be relieved by slowly stretching the muscle and massaging it with an oil containing a stimulant and an analgesic.

Vulneraries stimulate cell growth and thus speed up tissue repair. Choose herbs like aloe vera and chamomile to treat any muscle and tendon damage.

Stimulants or rubefacients dilate small blood vessels to stimulate circulation and relieve pain. Use rosemary, eucalyptus, and clove to relieve rheumatic aches and pains.

Analgesics help to reduce pain through external application. Use St. John's wort, lavender, clove, peppermint, and chamomile for pain caused by chronic fatigue, recently overextended muscles, or flu.

Anti-inflammatories fight inflammation. For pain due to recently overextended muscles or accompanied by redness and swelling, use chamomile, St. John's wort, and lavender.

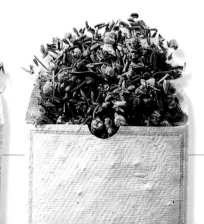
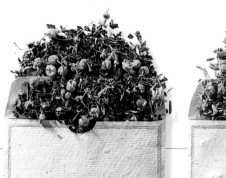

Infused St. John's wort oil is deep red in color, despite the fact that the flowers of the plant are bright yellow. St. John's wort contains a red pigment, hypericin, which is extracted from the plant by infusing the fresh herb in olive oil in direct sunlight. Hypericin carries the anti-inflammatory and pain-relieving properties for which St. John's wort is so popular.

very effective way of easing aching muscles that accompany influenza. You should not take a whole-body bath while running a fever, so a footbath is the ideal alternative.

BACK MASSAGE FOR MUSCLE TENSION

Back pain can range from mild discomfort to severe and debilitating pain. It can also lead to other disorders such as headaches and pains in the legs and neck. Muscle tension in the back is commonly a result of stress, bad posture, or overstraining, and a chronic backache can result in many other muscular and mobility problems.

Before you receive massage for back pain, be sure that your condition is not caused by anything more serious than a muscle spasm or tension. It might, for example, be a prolapsed disc. If in doubt, consult your doctor, who will be able to advise you if massage is a suitable therapy for your condition.

If you are giving rather than receiving a back massage, make sure that the person being massaged is warm and comfortable, then apply a hot compress over the painful area to loosen and prepare the muscles. Remove the compress before you begin to massage, and use a liberal amount of oil so your hands glide easily over the skin.

With smooth, flowing strokes, work gently over the whole of the back and hips. You may increase the pressure of your strokes gradually, taking care not to cause any additional discomfort. If the person receiving the massage feels uncomfortable at any time, the massage should be discontinued.

MAKING YOUR OWN MASSAGE OIL FOR MUSCLE ACHES

An infused oil made from fresh St. John's wort flowers (available from herbal suppliers) has anti-inflammatory and pain-relieving properties that make it an excellent massage oil for pain relief. The addition of certain essential oils can enhance and complements its therapeutic qualities. Both chamomile and lavender have antispasmodic properties, which relax muscles and help to relieve tension when used in massage. Clove oil has a strong analgesic action and is very good for muscular pain.

Ingredients

250 ml (1⅛ cups) St. John's wort infused oil (do not use the essential oil, which can irritate skin if applied directly to it)
5 drops lavender essential oil
1 drop chamomile essential oil
2 drops clove essential oil

1 *Pour the St. John's wort oil into a clean bottle. Slowly add the essential oils, one at a time. When all the oils have been added, close the bottle tightly and shake well to blend the essential oils with the base oil.*

2 *During a massage, shake the bottle well before each use. Apply the oil liberally and work it into the skin.*

A dark glass bottle will help to keep oils at full strength.

3 *It is a good idea for the recipient to have a bath or shower before a massage to warm and loosen the muscles. Begin by massaging the area gently, increasing the strength of your strokes as you proceed.*

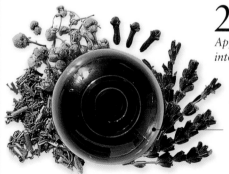

NERVOUS DISORDERS

Herbal remedies can offer gentle but effective relief from the nervous, emotional, and physical tensions that crop up in life from time to time.

Left unattended, problems such as insomnia and depression, which may result from the stresses of living, can become life-changing disorders. It is important to deal with minor problems of day-to-day life before they become too challenging or even defeating. Chronic pain can also lead to emotional ill health.

ANXIETY AND INSOMNIA

Work and family pressures produce anxiety and insomnia in many people. Symptoms include general restlessness, palpitations, lack of concentration, and unspecified fears.

Many herbal remedies used to treat anxiety relax and strengthen the nervous system at the same time. Gentle nerve tonics such as chamomile, lemon balm, wood betony, and skullcap should be used over a long period to obtain the best results. They may be taken as a tea or tincture.

Stronger sedative herbs are suitable for times of acute restlessness or insomnia. Valerian, passionflower, and hops taken as tinctures or added to a warm (not hot) bath help to promote sleep. Hops should not be used by people who suffer from depression.

DEPRESSION

The symptoms of depression include anxiety, insomnia, loss of appetite, and lack of energy. A person with depression usually has vast feelings of hopelessness.

The herb of choice to treat depression is St. John's wort, a traditional remedy for nervous disorders. Recent clinical studies have also found St. John's wort to be an effective antidepressant if taken internally over long periods. Scientists in Germany compare the action of St. John's wort to that of monoamine oxidase inhibitors, a group of conventional drugs that stimulate the brain and are currently used in treating depression. St. John's wort combines well with other nerve tonics, such as lemon balm, rosemary, and skullcap, and can be taken as a tincture or a tea in standard doses over long periods of time. One caution: St. John's wort can make the skin more sensitive to sunlight; therefore people who have fair skin should avoid long exposure to the sun while taking it.

STRESS

Prolonged or particularly high levels of stress cause many of today's illnesses, as well as reducing the body's ability to ward off infections and depleting energy levels. Unlike a virus or bacteria, the fundamental cause of stress can be difficult to diagnose, and its effects vary from person to person. This makes treatment difficult, but herbs can be used to boost both the physical and emotional responses to stress.

Recurrent infections

Physical and emotional stress can weaken the immune system and result in recurrent infections, such as cold sores and upper respiratory infections. Echinacea is one of the best-known and most researched herbs for boosting the immune system. It increases the body's production of white blood cells to fend off infections. Echinacea should be taken only for acute conditions. Taken over long periods, it can overstimulate the immune system and further deplete resources. For recurrent infections, take 1 teaspoon of the tincture up to four times a day as soon as symptoms appear. Take it only until the infection has cleared and then discontinue using the herb.

Mugwort may be taken in the same way as echinacea to treat acute infections, but it is very bitter and must be used in small doses—5 to 10 drops of tincture up to four times a day—until the condition improves. (Avoid mugwort during pregnancy.)

Emotional relief
Emotional problems can have many triggers, including stress and the difficulties of long-term physical pain. Holistic herbal treatment looks at the physical and emotional aspects of a problem at the same time and attempts to relieve both of them.

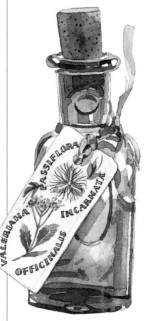

EMOTIONAL PAIN RELIEF Tincture of willow bark taken internally has mild analgesic properties, as do many other sedative herbs, like passionflower and valerian. All help to support the action of external preparations used to relieve physical symptoms, such as pain.

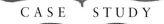

An Insomniac

Insomnia disrupts important physical patterns and often leaves the sufferer disorientated and drained of energy. These effects can lead to further sleep disruption if pressures from work and home build up. Herbal remedies and simple lifestyle changes can help to restore a natural and healthy sleeping pattern.

William is 39 years old and married to Pam. They have two children and recently moved to a new house. William runs his own business, and keeping it going, as well as coping with the move, has been extremely stressful. He regularly works late and on weekends and eats on the move, although he has his main meal when he comes home at night, often around 10 P.M. He is finding it increasingly difficult to get to sleep and often wakes in the early hours of the morning. He drinks frequent cups of black coffee throughout the day to give him energy but is having increasing difficulty concentrating on work. His relationship with Pam and the children has begun to suffer, as he finds it harder and harder to keep an even temper.

WHAT WILLIAM SHOULD DO

William should create a more reasonable work schedule, leaving time for his family and relaxation. A warm bath in the evening with lavender oil added to it will help him relax.

William should also try to eat his dinner earlier in the evening. Going to bed on a full stomach may be adding to his sleeping difficulties. He should cut down on caffeinated drinks and try herbal teas, particularly mild nerve tonics, to help him relax. A good combination is chamomile, lemon balm, wood betony, and rosemary in equal parts. He could also try taking 2 teaspoons of a tincture containing stronger sedative herbs, such as valerian, passionflower, and hops, half an hour before going to bed.

Action Plan

WORK
Reorganize your working day. Long working hours are not necessarily productive and often cause additional stress.

LIFESTYLE
Avoid heavy evening meals and particularly try not to eat after 8 P.M. Make time to exercise each day, if possible, and take up some form of relaxation.

HEALTH
Take herbal teas and tonics to help relax the body and calm mental and emotional states before bedtime.

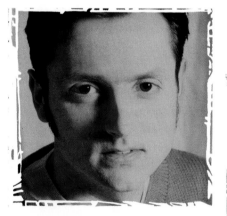

WORK
Overwork and irregular working hours can upset natural sleeping patterns.

LIFESTYLE
Eating irregularly and having little time for relaxation or exercise can lead to sleeplessness.

HEALTH
Excessive caffeine can disrupt sleep and cause health problems in the long term.

HOW THINGS TURNED OUT FOR WILLIAM

William is now much more disciplined about his working hours—though he still works on weekends occasionally—and enjoys having more time to spend with his children. He replaced most of his coffee with herbal tea, which he finds soothing, and he believes it has helped reduce his overall stress levels. He started to sleep better after three weeks of taking the herbs and has been able to reduce the sedative tincture to 1 teaspoon every other night.

PROBLEMS OF AGING

Growing old affects physical and mental abilities and reduces strength and immunity to illnesses. This can lead to general poor health and chronic disorders affecting mobility and vitality.

Several disorders are widely considered to be simply the normal, natural results of increasing age. Forgetfulness, loss of concentration, and cold hands and feet caused by poor circulation are common examples of age-related problems. The only difficulty with this attitude is that some people may allow their faculties to degenerate because they think it is inevitable. For many signs of aging—for example, circulation and joint problems—there are various courses of action that can prevent decline.

CIRCULATORY PROBLEMS

It is well known that circulatory disorders are most common among the middle-aged and elderly. These emerge in two main ways as the heart muscle becomes weaker. First, the amount of blood that is pumped through the system with each heartbeat lessens; second, the rate at which the heart beats increases to fulfill the body's needs. Other age-related changes involving the heart include atherosclerosis, raised blood pressure, and a thickening around the valves of the heart.

To keep these disorders at bay, it may help to investigate the cardiovascular properties of herbs. Some have proved highly effective in promoting adequate circulation and maintaining healthy blood pressure.

Angelica, juniper, and cayenne stimulate arterial circulation, and are often used to treat cold hands and feet, chilblains, and some more serious circulatory disorders. Cayenne pepper is also a useful heart stimulant. Angelica and juniper should be taken as tinctures, 2 to 5 millileters three times a day, but avoid juniper if you suffer from weak kidneys. Cayenne can be taken as a tincture, 3 to 4 drops, or a powder, a small pinch taken in a tea three to six times a day.

The leaves of the ginkgo tree (*Ginkgo biloba*) are known to improve circulation of the blood. Taken internally as a tincture, tea, or capsule, ginkgo can help to reduce tiredness, improve concentration and memory, and give energy levels a boost. It is a slow-acting remedy and should be taken three times a day for at least six weeks before improvements begin to show.

Circulatory tonics like hawthorn and rosemary gently strengthen and regulate the function of the heart. When combined with ginkgo, they can help improve circulation to all parts of the body. While hawthorn is best taken as a tincture—2 to 4 millileters three times a day—rosemary makes a pleasant infusion, which should be drunk every day. Both herbs can be used over long periods of time with no side effects.

Ginseng has long been used as a tonic for old age. Not only does it strengthen the circulation and improve the body's overall resistance to disease, but it also stimulates the central nervous system. It can be either

---

CHRONIC FATIGUE

A general lack of energy and chronic fatigue may become more common with advancing age. There are many herbs that can help relieve fatigue, but their use should be part of general lifestyle changes to boost energy.

Ginseng is an adaptogen, used to reduce stress and increase physical performance and mental abilities. It should be taken in small doses—1 gram per day, well chewed, or 10 drops of tincture twice a day—and for not more than three months, to prevent side effects such as insomnia, headaches, and restlessness.

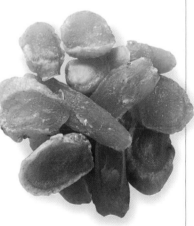

CRYSTALLINE SUPER BOOST
Ginseng is usually available dried or crystallized because the fresh plant is protected.

chewed raw—1 gram daily—or made into a tincture—10 drops once or twice every day. There is some evidence to suggest that ginseng should not be taken by people who have high blood pressure, and it may cause headaches if taken in large doses. Ginseng combines well, however, with other tonic herbs such as rosemary, mugwort, skullcap, and wood betony.

ARTHRITIS

Rheumatoid arthritis is caused by the body's immune system reacting against the body itself. Although it can strike at any age, it is particularly common among the elderly. The condition is characterized by swellings and deformities of the joints, which can become very hot and painful. Osteoarthritis, caused by the wearing away of joints, leads to stiffness and pain. Internal treatment is the same for both types.

Flushing out toxins and waste products through the kidneys and liver is an important part of herbal treatment for arthritis. Alterative herbs like celery, dandelion, and burdock help keep the body free from the toxins that contribute to the condition. These herbs are best taken as a tincture or a tea in standard doses over an extended period of time to achieve a cumulative effect.

Before aspirin became available as a drug, herbalists used the bark of the willow tree (see page 119) to relieve the pain of arthritis. Willow bark is most effective when

SOOTHING ARTHRITIS
For external treatment, apply a cold compress over a hot and painful arthritic joint. The addition of a few drops of essential oil of peppermint will enhance the cooling effect. Clinical trials in Germany have found that peppermint also has a strong analgesic action if applied externally, which will provide additional pain relief. For cold, stiff joints, use rubefacient massage oils, such as rosemary or thyme. An herbal hand bath can also be very beneficial for relieving arthritis pain.

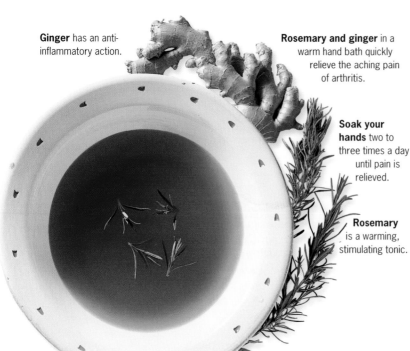

Ginger has an anti-inflammatory action.

Rosemary and ginger in a warm hand bath quickly relieve the aching pain of arthritis.

Soak your hands two to three times a day until pain is relieved.

Rosemary is a warming, stimulating tonic.

CAUTION
While celery seeds may be used with complete safety, the isolated essential oil (apiol) of celery is toxic and should be used with caution and never by pregnant women. Similarly, colchicum, recommended for gout, is a toxic plant that should be used only as recommended by a qualified practitioner. It can cause nausea, diarrhea, and vomiting, and must not be taken during pregnancy.

taken as a decoction—3 cups daily—or as a tincture—5 milliliters three times a day. Treatment with willow bark will take a few days to begin working.

The famous English herbalist Gerard wrote in 1597 that cabbage "is marvellous for the sinewes and joints." Fresh cabbage, lightly crushed and applied as a poultice to a painful joint, is an old folk remedy that is still used today. Cover the entire joint with a cabbage leaf and keep it in place with a clean cotton cloth. Apply a new leaf every 20 minutes until the pain has eased.

GOUT

A disease resulting from a buildup of uric acid in the body, gout causes painful inflammation and swelling of the joints and is most commonly found to affect the big toe.

The long-term treatment for gout is similar to that for arthritis, with a special emphasis on alterative herbs for the kidneys and liver, such as those mentioned for arthritis, above. A diet low in foods that contain purines is also important for successful long-term treatment. Gout sufferers should avoid sardines, anchovies, shellfish, red meat, and beans. Alcohol and stimulants like tea and coffee should also be excluded from the diet; they can be replaced by caffeine-free herbal teas or water.

Attacks of gout can be prevented and relieved with colchicine, an alkaloid extracted from autumn crocus (*Colchicum autumnale*, also known as meadow saffron), which lessens the buildup of uric acid in the body. However, colchicine is highly toxic and is available only by prescription. Poultices of cabbage leaves will also help to relieve the pain (see Arthritis, above).

INDEX

157

ACKNOWLEDGMENTS

Carroll & Brown Limited
would like to thank
Chelsea Physic Garden
Cosmetic Toiletry and Perfume
  Association, London
National Herbalists' Association of
  Australia, Morisset, NSW
Neal's Yard Remedies
Sacred Hoop Magazine
Weleda (UK) Ltd

Editorial assistants
Sharon Freed
Simon Warmer

DTP design
Elisa Merino

Photograph sources
  8 Kings College School of
      Medicine/Department of
      Surgery/SPL
 10 Science Photo Library
 11 Paul Biddle/SPL
 12 Dr Morley Read/SPL
 13 Bridgeman Art Library
 18 (Top) Heather Angel,
      (Bottom) David Murray/C & B
 19 Oxford Scientific Films
 20 (All) Bridgeman Art Library
 21 (All) Bridgeman Art Library
 22 (Left) Mary Evans Picture
      Library, (Right) Giraudon/
      Bridgeman Art Library
 23 (All) Bridgeman Art Library
 25 Mary Evans Picture Library
 27 Science Photo Library
 28 Tony Stone Images
 30 David Murrary/C & B
 35 The C W Daniel Co Ltd
 43 Andrew Syred/SPL
 44 Tony Stone Images
 56 *Chatterton*, Henry Wallis/Tate
      Gallery Publications
 58 (Top) Michael Strobing/Oxford
      Scientific Films, (Centre) John
      Glover/ Garden Picture Library,

(Bottom) G. A. Maclean/Oxford
Scientific Films
 59 (Top) Geoff Kidd/Oxford
      Scientific Films, (Foxglove and
      Henbane) David Murray/C & B,
      (Bottom) Frithjof Skibbe/Oxford
      Scientific Films
 60 (Top) Mike Slater/Oxford
      Scientific Films, (Lobelia) Ron
      Bass/Botanical Collection Ltd.,
      (Bittersweet) DeniBrown/Oxford
      Scientific Films, (Bottom) Tim
      Shepherd/Oxford Scientific films
 68 Henk Dijkman/Garden Picture
      Library
 70 Tim Griffith/Garden Picture
      Library
 71 Wellcome Institute Library
 87 (Bottom) Bridgeman Art Library
 89 Elizabeth Rice/Bridgeman Art
      Library
 90 (Top) Elizabeth Rice/Bridgeman
      Art Library
 92 (Bottom) Elizabeth Rice/
      Bridgeman Art Library
 94 (Top) Elizabeth Rice /Bridgeman
      Art Library
 94 (Bottom) Bridgeman Art Library
 97 Bridgeman Art Library
104 (Bottom) Elizabeth Rice/
      Bridgeman Art Library
107 (Top) Elizabeth Rice/Bridgeman
      Art Library
108 (Bottom) Elizabeth Rice/
      Bridgeman Art Library
111 (Bottom) Elizabeth Rice/
      Bridgeman Art Library
112 (Bottom) Elizabeth Rice/
      Bridgeman Art Library
113 (Bottom) Elizabeth Rice/
      Bridgeman Art Library
114 (Bottom) Elizabeth Rice/
      Bridgeman Art Library
115 (Top) Elizabeth Rice/Bridgeman
      Art Library
118 (Bottom) Elizabeth Rice/
      Bridgeman Art Library
118 (Top) Bridgeman Art Library,
119 (Top) Elizabeth Rice/Bridgeman

Art Library
120 Elizabeth Rice/Bridgeman
      Art Library
121 (Top) Elizabeth Rice/Bridgeman
      Art Library
124 (Bottom) Bridgeman Art Library
126 (Top) Elizabeth Rice/Bridgeman
      Art Library
127 (Top) Bridgeman Art Library
129 (Top) Elizabeth Rice/Bridgeman
      Art Library
130 (Bottom) Elizabeth Rice/
      Bridgeman Art Library
132 (Top) Elizabeth Rice/Bridgeman
      Art Library

Botanical illustrators
Pam Baldaro
Angelika Elsebach
Sarah Fuller
Will Giles
Sandra Pond
Ann Winterbotham

Illustrators
John Geary
Nicola Gregory
Sarah Venus
Anthea Whitworth

Photographic assistants
M-A Hugo
Mark Langridge

Hair and make-up
Kim Menzies

Picture research
Sandra Schneider

Research
Steven Chong

Index
Laura Price